# BREAKING OUT

## of Environmental Illness

**ESSENTIAL READING FOR PEOPLE WITH
CHRONIC FATIGUE SYNDROME,
ALLERGIES & CHEMICAL SENSITIVITIES**

Robert Sampson, M.D. & Patricia Hughes, B.S.N.

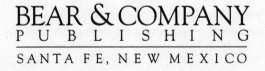

BEAR & COMPANY
PUBLISHING
SANTA FE, NEW MEXICO

LIBRARY OF CONGRESS CATALOGING-IN-PUBLICATION DATA

Sampson, Robert 1948-
    Breaking out of environmental illness : essential reading for people with chronic fatigue syndrome, allergies, and chemical sensitivities / Robert Sampson and Patricia Hughes.
        p. cm.
    Includes bibliographical references.
    ISBN 1-879181-41-X
    1. Sampson, Robert, 1948—Health.   2. Hughes, Patricia, 1954—Health.
3. Environmentally induced diseases—Patients—United States—Biography.
4. Chronic fatigue syndrome.   5. Allergy.   6. Environmental toxicology.
I. Hughes, Patricia, 1954- .   II. Title.
RB152.S26    1996
362. 1' 9698' 00922—dc2197-7512
[B]                    CIP

Copyright © 1997 by Robert Sampson and Patricia Hughes

Bear & Company, Inc.
Santa Fe, NM 87504-2860


Cover and interior design: Melinda Belter

Cover and interior illustrations: copyright © Francene Hart

Editing: Sonya Moore and Sarah Zarbock

Printed in the United States of America by BookCrafters, Inc.,
on totally chlorine free (TCF) paper with environmentally safe soy ink.


9 8 7 6 5 4 3 2 1

# Praise for the Authors' Healing Work

Dr. Sampson and Patricia Hughes were delightful to work with. They played a very significant role in my journey to wellness. I tried many different holistic forms of healing. However, journeying with them was a unique healing experience. They were unusual in that they had medical backgrounds and had suffered very debilitating illnesses. When I started working with Dr. Sampson and Patricia, I myself was suffering from severe CFIDS. I am now recovered enough to work as a certified herbalist and have dedicated myself to helping others to wellness using many of the tools I learned from them. I will forever be grateful for all their caring and sharing.

*Noreen Pray, herbalist*

Just when my life had become unbearable and my future unthinkable, I met Dr. Sampson and Patricia Hughes; and they began to guide me out of the jungle of environmental illness. In many cases, the traditional and alternative therapies which are available are unable to penetrate this serious and disabling condition.

Dr. Sampson has looked deeper and sought answers from within the psyche. He is not only my doctor, but also a great teacher. He is showing me that although my illness was triggered by a toxic chemical exposure, there is much I can do to heal the deeper layers of my body. He uses energy balancing, chakra clearing, thought clearing, and the Nambudripad Allergy Elimination Technique (NAET). I realize now that he is helping me heal on a much deeper level that has been sadly neglected by the traditional medical system, and Patricia has a profound sense of how our lives are influenced by our thoughts and our surroundings.

My visits with Dr. Sampson and Patricia Hughes are transformational. I become renewed and enlightened by their words and knowledge. Through their hard work and personal lessons, the path is being cleared for others. Until now, there has been very little success in treating environmental illness. Dr. Sampson and Patricia Hughes bring new hope for the environmentally ill everywhere.

*L.S., teacher*

After suffering with many allergies all my life and spending four-and-a-half years bedridden with Chronic Immune Dysfunction Syndrome (CFIDS), I found the energy therapies which Dr. Sampson used (including NAET) instrumental in starting me on the path to providing my body with what it needed to heal.

*Diane Bocchino*

I was diagnosed with Chronic Fatigue Syndrome, or chronic EBV, over a decade ago. After consulting with some of the best infectious disease doctors and considering numerous treatments, it became apparent that they could not help me. I have used numerous alternative treatments; Dr. Sampson's use of NAET has had the most positive effect on my health. My blood pressure, which was unstable, stabilized; and my pulse has become more consistently normal. I have gained stamina and strength, and a greater sense of well-being.

Although I am not cured, I am reaching new levels of health which I thought were impossible to achieve.

*Anonymous*

Working with Robert and Patricia was an incredibly enriching and transformative experience for me. I feel blessed to have found them on my journey. With a unique and nurturing approach, Robert and Patricia helped me to overcome my battle with chronic physical conditions, as well as debilitating negative thought patterns. Under their guidance, I was able to reach a place of much greater physical, mental, emotional, and spiritual health. I have attained a sense of peace, joy, wisdom, acceptance, and personal fulfillment that I never knew I could have. They have been extremely helpful in facilitating my ability to manifest that which I truly desire in my life.

*Alison Leeds Puth, teacher*

Robert and Patricia combine their medical training with a personal understanding of environmental illness and years of exploring new techniques for healing. The result is an effective mix of therapies they can draw upon to address this baffling illness.

In session, they are intuitive healers and teachers who show deep respect for where I am and artfully challenge me to take the next step. After years of illness, my stamina is growing and so is my faith that I can heal.

*Anonymous*

Robert and Patricia heal on a level that is much deeper than the physical. When I leave their office, I feel an incredible sense of well-being. Over the months the effect has become cumulative. On a level that is more profound than healing Multiple Chemical Sensitivity Syndrome, they have given me a sense of total well-being greater than I have ever felt before.

Robert and Patricia's work is not limited to their treatment but includes massive amounts of information from their personal experiences and many exercises and techniques to allow me to continue the healing process on my own. This feels very empowering.

*B.Z.*

When I first started treatments with Robert and Patricia, I was unable to eat most foods except for some proteins, two grains, and some vegetables. I would even have allergic reactions just walking through a supermarket! I responded well and was able to start expanding my diet almost immediately. After several months I was able to eat all foods once again with no restrictions. I have also noticed other health benefits such as normal (rather than low) blood pressure and a consistent, overall increase in energy.

*Mary S., receptionist*

Throughout my life I have searched for a truly effective way to address what had become debilitating environmental and food allergies. That search took me through an array of methods such as various medications, limiting exposure, restrictive diets, allergy shots, vitamins, homeopathic drops, and, of course, my last resort—to continue to suffer. The work I have done with Robert and Patricia has not only been enjoyable and enlightening but, most importantly, has truly worked! For the last eighteen months my allergies have been reduced by 80 to 90 percent. I can now eat and play outside without severe symptoms. Thank you.

*Gary Lospaluto*
*copresident, Collaborative Action Associates*

Sometimes people try things out of desperation that they would not ordinarily consider. That is how I came to meet Robert and Patricia.

In 1989 I began a personal battle with depression. Over the years I tried all traditional methods of treatment with no reliable success. Last year, completely exhausted from this struggle to survive, I came very close to taking my own life. The reason I didn't is because a friend, who also struggles with depression, told me about an alternative approach. My desperation gave me the courage to make an appointment with Robert and Patricia.

I still can't explain what they did. Many times I had to work hard to suspend my beliefs in order just to accept the positive benefits of their methods. Sometimes I'd just want to laugh outright at a particularly weird treatment. Often I cried because they were helping me reach deeply sad places in my life that were full of unspent tears. I came away from each meeting feeling better and better.

After awhile, I stopped trying to figure out the whats and the whys. All that was important was that something very good was happening, and I was beginning to feel alive again. Since then, my husband, my teenager, and my two-year-old have all benefitted from meetings with Robert and Patricia.

I have the highest regard and admiration for the breadth of their knowledge, their professionalism, and their caring. I am so grateful that I came to know them and experience their healing.

*Elaine Z.L.*

# Praise for <u>Breaking Out of Environmental Illness</u>

"*Breaking Out of Environmental Illness* presents in exceedingly readable fashion two courageous souls' responses to the ultimate health crises: allergy to the environment. Their story of emerging from crises to form a healing relationship with body, emotions, mind, and spirit, all in the context of love for our home planet, deserves our fullest attention and respect. Many thanks to Robert and Patricia for articulating their struggle and their triumph. In a very real sense their journey represents all of our journeys as we enter the twenty-first century."
　　*—Steven L. Schatz, MA, director, Center For Music and Imagery*

"Through a well-written and captivating narrative, Robert Sampson and Patricia Hughes have clearly described the nightmare of environmental illness. Their story illustrates the extremely important point that the "true" answers to breaking out of chronic illness lie deep within us, not in the external world. Therefore, this book is a 'must-read' for anyone who wants to overcome a serious chronic illness. I intend to ask all of my patients who are suffering with a long-term illness to read this book."
　　*—Mark Fradkin, Dipl. Ac., L.Ac.*

"*Breaking Out of Environmental Illness* is a fascinating story of a shamanic journey—getting to the bottom of despair, of hopelessness and helplessness only to come out (albeit at times kicking and screaming) on the other side of surrender. On one level it's a story of how Patricia and Robert got to heal their environmental illness, yet on a deeper level, their story provides an exciting illustration of how we create our own reality."
　　*—Mira A. Furth, M.Ed., cofounder, Changeworks,*
　　*enterprise for education and healing, Andover, MA*

"As we read of Robert and Patricia's experiences we find they reflect the lives of many persons we serve at The Living Source. The book is true, stimulating, and hard to put down."
　　*—James M. Summers, Ph.D., consultant,*
　　*and Nancy T. Summers, president, The Living Source*

"This exciting and powerful book is enthralling, informative, and I couldn't stop reading it. The authors' journey is definitely one worth sharing."
　　*—Angela C. Grattaroti, LICSW*

Dedicated to The Goddess
as She returns to Earth now, and
to those choosing to receive Her

# Contents

# Acknowledgments

We wish to thank Barbara Hand Clow and Gerry Clow as well as the other staff at Bear & Company for their superb efforts in bringing this book through the publication process in a rapid and timely manner.

We thank our guides and teachers from both Seen and Unseen realms for their help, assistance, and support.

We thank our many friends, too many to list completely, who both listened to our doubts and fears and gave us support. These include Les, Thom, Christine, Amy, Gary, Melissa, Mira, Lauren, Adriana, Sheila.

We thank the many beings from the Nature Kingdom for their support and instruction including the Devas, the Ants, the Deer, the Baby Birds, and the many other animals who brought us messages.

We give special thanks to Mary Jonaitis, Pat Balzer, and Sheila Simon for their efforts in connecting us to sources of wisdom which gave new directions to our healing process and for their continual willingness to open to the Unknown.

Lastly, we wish to honor one another for loving and supporting each other through this extraordinary transformational process and through the writing of this book.

# Special Notice to the Reader

Each person's healing will take him or her on a unique journey. Environmental illness, chronic fatigue syndrome, and related disorders can be particularly puzzling and difficult health problems. Although this book was written by a physician and a nurse and discusses various techniques which they used in their own healing process, *it is not meant to give specific recommendations or advice for the diagnosis or treatment of particular illnesses.* Experience has shown that healing often involves a collaborative effort between an individual and one or more health-care practitioners which activates and encourages the individual's own innate healing powers.

Robert Sampson, M.D., & Patricia Hughes, B.S.N.

# Breaking Out
## of
# Environmental Illness

# Patricia's Introduction

I was very ill and very frightened when I met Robert in 1989. At the age of thirty-four I had given up on a social life. All my time was spent working, buying and preparing food, making my apartment safe, and recovering from exposures to chemicals. It was becoming increasingly difficult to tolerate the coronary intensive care unit where I worked as a nurse. I was beginning to realize I would have to quit my job. But what would I do to support myself? My world was becoming smaller and smaller in spite of my special diet, herbal and nutritional supplements, and environmental controls outside of work. Moving to my mother's home in North Carolina was not an option. I could not tolerate her fully carpeted house, let alone deal with all the ramifications of having to admit I could no longer work.

Religion was not a big focus in my family. My father never spoke to us about his religious convictions. My mother was disillusioned with the Catholic Church, and exposed us to the teachings only out of a feeling of obligation. The resentment and lack of connection to the church was communicated nonverbally, and when I learned the definition of the word "agnostic" in my late teens, I realized I was one. The innate knowledge I had held as a child, that I was protected by a loving, benevolent, unseen force I could feel over my shoulder, had been lost.

Robert, on the other hand, had a deep connection to God from early on. He was raised in a Christian family. He picked up a book on yoga and began to practice when he was twelve. When I met him, he'd been meditating daily for twenty years. His apartment was full of statues and pictures of Shiva, Kali, Ganesha, Buddha, Yogananda, Christ, the Mother Mary, angels, dolphins, Pele, and sacred Chinese figures. He talked of acupuncture, Taoist teachings, tai chi, and Iron Shirt Qi Gong. It was all new to me. When he heard me describe him as a "New Age guy" to my sister, he became indignant, saying these things had been an integral part of his life long before the phrase "New Age" was coined. I thought he was really weird.

After two months of dating (if you call walking on the beach and eating my specially prepared meals dating), I ended our relationship. A therapist I had been seeing was pushing me to examine and deal with a new aspect of the abuse I had experienced as a child, telling me I was a post-traumatic stress survivor. My response was to feel totally contaminated and damaged, and unable to be in a relationship. And Robert was just too strange.

Three months later, during a six-week sick leave from work related to my environmental illness, I found myself praying to God. This was not something I did often. I was bordering on atheism. But I was at a total loss. I just could not do this alone anymore, and I was unwilling to consider disability. Tears streaming down my face, I prayed for a partner who would understand my illness, be willing to tolerate my limitations, and maybe even help me get well.

You can bet I was shocked to hear a loud, clear voice say "You've already met him." Robert's smile flashed before my eyes. I looked up toward the heavens. "Robert?" I asked in disbelief. "Yes" came the reply. "But he's so weird!" I complained. "That's him, my Dear" was the response, and the end of the communication, for the time being. Still, I did not contact him. Coincidentally (or not), we ran into each other four months later. Thus began our journey together.

For over fifteen years, Robert had known he was going to write an unusual, ground-breaking book, though it was not clear what it would be about. He realized in 1991 that the book was about our healing process. But he thought of it as HIS book, and was slow to let me join him in the writing. He wrote the first two parts essentially alone. Most of it poured out of him. He would read it to me, ask for input, and get irritated with my response. I would get angry and refuse to continue the conversation. And so it went, intermittently, for three-and-a-half years.

A major theme in my healing involved becoming willing to express myself fully in the moment. Having learned early in life that safety was had by being quiet and staying out of the way, this was quite a process for me. But as I did so, I found I had a lot to say. After two years studying the psychospiritual dynamics of the masculine and feminine, I was ready. I chose to go around Robert's irritation and resistance to my input. Instead of letting him read to me, I picked up the manuscript and started editing. The editing turned into writing. Robert was surprised by how much he liked it. After years of stop and go, push and pull, and feeble, disconnected attempts to work together, suddenly we found ourselves working in a cocreative flow that delighted, challenged, and energized both of us.

Robert's writing style is concise and factual. He is great at remembering events and dates, and structuring the story (the masculine flow). My style is flowing, rambling, chaotic. I brought in the emotions and the personal, intimate details (the feminine flow). It took a lot for Robert to be willing to allow himself to be exposed in that manner. And it was interesting to try to combine the two styles into one cohesive story.

The process of writing this book has been much like the process of our relationship. For a long time we wondered why we were together, and didn't really know how to connect. Yet we were clear we wanted to stay together. Whenever I questioned that decision, something or someone always came along and reminded me of the special nature of our relationship.

It was my prayers to find a partner who would love and accept me in my deepest moments of despair that brought Robert back to me, even though I had rejected him, and eventually brought me my healing. In spite of the fact that I often think he was put on this planet to drive me crazy, I have come to realize that I will know myself and touch Divinity through honoring the sacredness of my relationship with Robert. And it is through the unfolding of this relationship that I have been able to begin to connect to my purpose, and to be of service. For this I am eternally grateful.

As we worked on the epilogue, I found that talking and writing about the masculine and feminine brought me great joy and excitement. I had to put a lid on it, or we would never have finished this book. We are considering writing a second book on that topic, soon. In the meantime, it is my sincere wish that this story will serve to inspire others and offer help and hope to those seeking healing.

# Robert's Introduction

Imagine a world where everything around you makes you sick. Your food, clothing, and shelter produce symptoms that may affect any organ in your body. Even low levels of chemicals that do not affect other people trigger reactions in you. Your life becomes a constant struggle to protect yourself from toxins that are everywhere around you. This is the world of someone with environmental illness. *Breaking Out of Environmental Illness* tells the story of how Patricia and I became trapped in that world and how we liberated ourselves from it. While both of our professional backgrounds are in health care, nothing in our training prepared us for what we experienced with environmental illness or gave us the tools to overcome it. Patricia, who worked in critical care nursing, became progressively more ill over many years until by 1990 she spent all of her time fighting to make it through the day and to keep her job. I am a psychiatrist whose illness began abruptly in July 1990 after being exposed to new carpet. This book, which has three parts, starts with that episode and is written from my perspective.

The first part describes our imprisonment in environmental illness. Prior to our meeting, Patricia had become steadily more sensitive and fatigued despite following the route of avoidance, desensitization, and nutritional support advocated by many holistic physicians and clinical ecologists. The sudden onset of my illness propelled us together as we looked for ways to get well. In spite of continuous efforts to avoid toxins, we became sicker and sicker. We were too sensitive to tolerate the antigen drops, herbs, and homeopathic remedies that are frequently used in alternative treatments of environmental illness.

The second part details our plight as our sensitivities continued to worsen. We put all our energies into creating a "safe house," but to no avail. By spring of 1991 we could not tolerate the inside of the house and had to sleep outdoors in a tent. Searching beyond holistic and alternative medicine, we discovered several energetic healing methods that helped temporarily; but we could not sustain the improvement. We kept hunting for a way to escape the living death that had engulfed us.

The third part chronicles what happened when we shifted our focus from feeling victimized by our symptoms to honoring them as communications from our bodies about various structures we had created in our lives which did not support us. Once we opened to this process, our healing took a totally different direction. We had to let go of everything we had created in our lives that was not truly nourishing for us: how we viewed our symptoms, what would alleviate them, how we were supposed to be, how we would make a living, what was and was not possible for us. Over eighteen months we healed our chemical sensitivities. This was not an easy process, but there was no other choice. Failure was not an option. We are happy to say we accomplished our goal of regaining our health and since then have far exceeded our expectations.

This book also includes a glossary and an appendix. The glossary contains definitions for words that we came across in our illness and recovery which may be unfamiliar to the reader. The appendix includes some of the energetic self-care techniques which we used in our recovery and insights we gained into the healing process.

We write from the perspective of having overcome environmental illness. For those readers with whom this book resonates we encourage you to use it as a vehicle to accelerate your own healing. For those who find the ideas contained herein difficult to accept, we understand your response. We had initial resistance to many of the ideas presented in part three. At times we became enraged by suggestions that such a process would help us. Ultimately, however, by letting ourselves explore the creative forces in a world outside the realm of conscious awareness, we found passage to freedom from our chemical sensitivities and a new sense of well-being we had not known was possible.

In the course of our healing we came to understand environmental illness in the broader context of massive changes that have been occurring on Earth since the late 1980s. Various visionaries and teachers throughout history have foreseen the period leading up to the year 2000 as a time of unprecedented change. Some have predicted cataclysmic destruction. Others envision an awakening of humanity to a totally new way of life with unlimited possibilities. We believe movement is already in progress to fulfill this latter prediction. This transition demands an end to the current way of living and the associated consciousness of separation from nature and from ourselves. We feel there is a relationship between the changes required for humanity to embody this new consciousness and the rising incidence of environmental illness, chronic fatigue syndrome, and related disorders noted in recent years.

For us environmental illness has been an amazing teacher, and we are grateful for the insights we have had as a result of our passage through it. Having gone into the depths of this illness, we know the pain it can entail and want to suggest a way out. We offer our very personal story of moving from being victimized by our health problems to embracing them as our personal wake-up call and an opening to undreamt of potentialities. We encourage others to entertain the same possibility for themselves. Dream big, ask Spirit for help, and remember to ask that it come to you in a loving and gentle way. You may be surprised by what you bring to yourself.

PART ONE

# The Prison

July 1990–March 1991

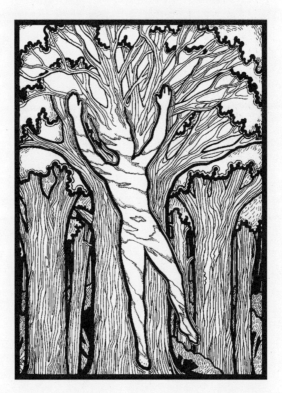

"Brer Rabbit pushed and he pulled and
he heaved and he ho'd. He kicked and he
squealed and he blew and he bawled but
the more he thrashed 'round the worse
off he got 'til he was so stuck up (in the
tar baby) he could scarcely move his
eyeballs."

*Song of the South*

# ONE

# Trapped

The pain had spread to my arms and legs. Now my chest started to hurt. Here I was in a retreat setting in the country, poised to learn about creating, and my body was going out of control. I had a hint of problems to come that morning in July 1990 on the first day of a five-day residential training. As I sat in the meeting room, I noticed aching in my right leg and thought it probably was a reaction to the new carpet on the floor. I was irritated by this intermittent discomfort; but it was tolerable, and I tried to ignore it. Little did I imagine that by evening I would fear for my life because of sudden, sharp chest pain.

Now, in a panic, I phoned my physician, Julia, and described my chest pain, muscle aching, and clouded thinking. I could sense her growing concern. Being a physician myself, I was all too aware of the implications of my chest pain, but as a psychiatrist it had been a long time since I had treated a patient with potentially life-threatening physical symptoms.

After completing my residency training in psychiatry and child psychiatry, I had studied a wide variety of alternative healing systems. With that background, I rarely consulted another doctor. When I found myself unable to alleviate a number of troubling symptoms even using alternative methods, I had sought the advice of Julia, a respected holistic physician.

When I told her about the new carpet in the conference room where I had spent most of the day, she shifted her focus. In light of my recently diagnosed sensitivity to several chemicals, she agreed that exposure to the carpet was the probable cause of these new symptoms.

I wanted to know what I should do. Was this life-threatening? How long would I feel like this? Would the pain go away? Julia reassured me that the symptoms would likely lessen once I recovered from this acute episode. The best thing to do was to avoid further exposure to the new carpet. She felt now that even the slightly older carpet in the bedroom might also bother me. She recommended I make alternative sleeping arrangements if I wanted to try to stay for the rest of the conference. If I were able to do that, I could see how I felt in the morning. The disappearance of symptoms would be a favorable indicator; their persistence would indicate a worse prognosis.

I trusted Julia's judgment and was glad to have spoken with her that evening. I took her advice and went outdoors to get away from the carpets. The night sky was filled with stars. In the past I would have enjoyed gazing at them. Now I only hoped the fresh air would relieve my symptoms. After about half an hour the sharp pain subsided. I was left with generalized achiness and clouded thinking.

I sought out the manager of the conference center to tell him about my dilemma. He had formerly maintained the center as an ashram and now rented it for personal growth workshops. When I informed him of what had happened, he responded with questions and doubt. He had never heard of carpet causing problems like mine. He asked how I could be sure it was the source of my symptoms. I described my discomfort as I sat in the room with the new carpet and told him of my conversation with my doctor who specialized in treating people with chemical sensitivities. My being a physician lent some credibility to what he otherwise seemed to feel was an unbelievable situation.

He asked what I wanted from him. With anxious determination I said I needed to sleep in a room that had no carpet. I wanted to find out whether being in a carpet-free setting would alleviate my symptoms so that I could continue with the workshop. Reluctantly, he agreed to see what he could do.

While he went to make arrangements, I spoke with the workshop leader. His work focused on helping people create what they wanted in their lives. After I related what had happened, he asked what I wanted to create in the workshop. I told him I wanted to complete the five days, but my health was my top priority. I was worried about how badly the carpet exposure had affected me. He suggested I wait to learn what the manager had arranged and to see how I felt the next morning.

As I awaited the manager's return, I remained outside in the cool night air. Never before had I appreciated fresh air so much. It was a relief to be outdoors away from the carpets. Shortly after nine-thirty the manager reappeared. He again emphasized that he had never heard of carpets making someone sick as I said his had made me. However, he would let me sleep in a nearby apartment with hardwood floors. I thanked him for his efforts and hoped this change would give me relief.

Taking no time to speak with the roommates I had met that morning, I quickly removed my belongings from the carpeted bedroom. My only thought was to escape the chemicals. I drove to a nearby building and walked up the stairs to a large apartment. The manager said it was usually rented to families attending conferences. Since it was free that week, I could stay there. I felt better away from the carpets but noticed a musty smell. I put the all-cotton sheets I had brought on the bed and removed as many items as possible from the room. Exhausted from the day's unexpected events, I fell into a deep sleep.

This temporary respite was broken early the next morning when the sun's rays awakened me. Many questions quickly filled my mind. Had all my symptoms gone away? Had I recovered my health? Was I going to be all right? As I became aware of my body and my mind, I had a sinking feeling. The intense muscle cramping and chest pain of the night before had disappeared, but I still had generalized muscle aching, cloudy thinking, and a sickening taste in my mouth.

Sadness filled me as I realized I no longer possessed the well-being I had even the morning before. In a state of denial I was unable to recognize or admit to myself how fragile my health had become. Amidst a confusing array of feelings I needed to decide whether or not to stay. I thought about what I had hoped to learn at the conference and about the twelve hundred dollars I had paid to attend. I was not willing to lose either the educational opportunity or the money. Considering all these factors, I decided to try to complete the remaining four days. Nevertheless, I knew I could not sit in the carpeted meeting room any more. As an alternative, I participated by listening from outside through a screened window.

This new arrangement was a mixed blessing. While providing relief from the carpet, it also exemplified the changed relationship I now had with my surroundings and would have for the next two years. I had gone to the workshop to join others from around the country in studying creating and consulting. Now I was staring from outside through a screened window trying to see and hear what was going on. I began to feel like a prisoner, looking in at events I wanted to be part of yet could not because something was wrong with my body.

Others had a variety of responses to this solution. The leader handled it well. He acknowledged and included me in discussions without putting undue emphasis on my being outside. Several participants were distressed by my separation from the group. Many appeared indifferent. Some interacted with me during breaks when they came outdoors to what had become my classroom. A few even thanked me for speaking out about my reactions. They said they were also having symptoms, such as headaches and drowsiness, which they had ignored until I spoke up.

Overall I interacted less with my classmates than I would have in the past. I ate outdoors as much as possible to minimize exposure to chemicals in the dining room rug. I avoided people wearing strong-smelling perfumes and colognes, which increased my muscle aching and clouded my thinking. Many times over the week I thought about how I was participating in the workshop from outside. A casual observer might have said I was separate and alienated from the others. Sometimes I felt that way. Although I would have enjoyed more involvement with them, any such interest had become secondary to keeping whatever health I still had and to lessening my reactivity to chemicals.

Fortunately, I did not have to cope with this dilemma alone. I made daily phone calls to Patty who knew well the difficulties I was just beginning to have. For more than four years she had suffered with extreme muscle aching, joint pain, weakness, headaches, fuzzy thinking, fatigue, and many other symptoms that I did not fully comprehend. Patty's physician had told her these symptoms were caused by environmental illness. Her doctor said that although Patty's health might improve, she would always be sensitive to chemicals. Patty explained to me that environmental illness involves overreactivity to numerous substances including foods, chemicals, and molds. She had tried to tell me about this disorder before, but I had no inkling of its profound impact until I experienced it myself. She assured me there were things that could be done to help with my reactions.

I had met Patty Hughes at a party sixteen months earlier. She was a registered nurse with years of experience in critical care. While we each rarely went to parties, we both felt compelled to go to that one. As I walked around the buffet table, I noticed this attractive woman whose presence seemed to call to me. I spoke with other people but my attention was repeatedly drawn to her. Finally, I knew I had to meet her so I went over and introduced myself. Once we started talking, it was clear we had a strong affinity for each other. The initial attraction was romantic, but there was also a not-yet-identified deeper connection. After the party we saw each other several times but then did not speak for months. In late 1989 through the efforts of a mutual friend we resumed contact.

After being diagnosed with environmental illness in 1988, Patty had begun changing her life in an attempt to regain her health. She had experienced improvement by changing her diet and creating a toxin-free home environment. She realized that constant exposure to chemicals in the coronary care unit where she worked hindered her recovery. As concern about AIDS increased, she found herself surrounded by more and more chemicals, including bleach and powerful cleaning agents. Whenever she put on the rubber gloves and the protective gear she was required to wear, she instantaneously experienced a burning, acrid sensation on her tongue and became intensely nauseous. Cotton glove liners offered limited relief. She had recently started working part-time in a holistic physician's office in an effort to find a less toxic job environment.

Patty recognized that urban air pollution was also a major problem for her. In pursuit of cleaner air she had moved to Newburyport, an hour's drive north of Boston on the Massachusetts coast. In early 1990 I invited her to stay at my apartment whenever she worked weekends. She had been able to manage the one-hour commute each way when she worked her usual ten-hour shift at Boston's Beth Israel Hospital, but the back-to-back twelve-hour weekend shifts she was required to work every third weekend were too much with the long drive. She accepted the invitation. On weekends when she was not working I often visited her in Newburyport. Now amidst this crisis brought on by the carpet at the conference center, Patty's support was very comforting.

The combination of spending as much time as possible outdoors and talking with Patty by phone allowed me to complete the training. Every noon I walked two miles to the beach and breathed in the refreshing ocean air. It was surprising how much my muscles relaxed. Back at the center, though, my muscles again became tight and achy.

At times I tried interacting with others by eating in the carpeted dining area. If I were there too long, my muscle aching worsened and the unpleasant taste in my mouth grew stronger. When Friday afternoon finally arrived, the leader and others gave me special recognition for staying to the end in spite of my symptoms. I felt grateful for having survived the carpet exposure and relieved to be able to leave.

During the hour's drive home my mind filled with questions. I had completed the five-day program but at what cost? What symptoms would remain? How much had my immune system been affected? Would I have to change my lifestyle? If so, how?

Even in the course of the trip, answers began to appear. I again experienced muscle aching and dizziness, which now seemed triggered by air pollution on the highway. Thinking about all the restrictions Patty lived with, I feared my life had been permanently changed and that my sensitivity to chemicals would mean persistent symptoms and limitation of my activities.

At first when I reached my apartment in Watertown, I was relieved to be back in the safety of my home, but with my heightened sensitivity to chemicals I soon began to view the apartment in a new light. The third-floor walkup had served me well for twelve years. Its convenient location allowed me to take advantage of educational and cultural opportunities in the Boston area. I had studied and practiced acupuncture and other forms of healing. My main job had been as psychiatrist at a nearby child guidance center. While I had previously felt fine healthwise in my apartment, I now noticed problems with muscle aching, coughing, confusion, and nausea. I wanted to know what was causing my symptoms and what would make them stop.

The next day I tried to see my doctor, but she was away. I met instead with her associate who began by reviewing my history. Intradermal allergy testing one month earlier revealed I was sensitive to many substances including dust, mites, molds, wheat, corn, milk, eggs, phenol, and alcohol. Based on my reaction to the carpet, she now tested me for formaldehyde by injecting varying dilutions of it under my skin. During this testing I developed tightness in my chest and throat, confusion, and muscle aching in my arms and hands just like I had at the conference. The results indicated definite sensitivity to formaldehyde. The aim of the testing was to find a dilution that would stop these symptoms. The doctor gave me drops to take under my tongue and told me to stay away from chemicals that bothered me. Essentially, I needed to avoid the chemicals of the twentieth century. I had become a person with environmental illness.

I did not fully understand what having environmental illness meant, but I knew I felt sick, and the sickness seemed related to exposure to chemicals, foods, and inhalants. My relationship to my life changed from living it to being its prisoner. Suddenly, I was intensely aware of being surrounded by numerous chemicals and other substances that were a source of danger.

Patty, who did dietary and lifestyle consultations for people with environmental illness, provided me with an abundant supply of information. She told me how I could lessen chemical exposures in my apartment. At her suggestion I removed insulated window shades, which I had purchased to conserve heat, and lived without shades over my windows. Bath towels now served as temporary curtains. I moved as many potentially toxic items as I could out of my bedroom, including my computer, its dustcovers, the computer stand, and bookcases. I bought special all-cotton covers, called "barrier cloths," for my bedding. The barrier cloths were made of tightly woven cotton to prevent exposure to dust mites and to the chemicals found in mattresses and pillows. These changes produced some lessening of my symptoms in the apartment.

Diet was another important consideration. For years I had eaten good quality food from the local whole foods supermarket. However, I had unintentionally fallen into a pattern limited to eating certain items including rice, vegetables, fish, chicken, fruit juices, soy drinks, cookies, and crackers. Given my sensitivity to many foods, I had the choice either to avoid them altogether or to eat them as part of a rotation diet. A rotation diet involves eating foods from a particular food family every four days. Having both followed one for years and taught clients to do so, Patty was well-versed in the rotation diet. She felt the diet had helped lessen her symptoms but complained about how time-consuming it was. She often spent four hours or more a day cooking.

With Patty's help, I organized foods I wanted to eat into a rotation. The most important ones to rotate were grains and proteins. The first day I ate wheat, chicken, and dairy, the second day rice and fish, the third day buckwheat, potatoes, and turkey, and the fourth day millet and other fish. Then the rotation started over again. I also rotated nuts, fruits, and vegetables. Being locked into this regimen was difficult at times, but I did my best. On the rotation diet I was pleased to notice the disappearance of sleepiness after lunch which I had been having for months. Patty told me drowsiness after meals is an indication of food allergy.

I asked myself what other symptoms of sensitivity to foods and chemicals had occurred previously without my recognizing them. I remembered the summer of 1989. Then during times of high humidity and high air pollution, I experienced pain in the joints of my hands. At forty-one years of age I told myself it was probably arthritis from getting older. When the symptoms disappeared on less humid days with less air pollution, I forgot about them.

I also recalled coughing, which began in November 1989 when I sublet an office for my private practice. Although at times I coughed so violently that my patients expressed concern about me, I made no connection between the office's new rug and furniture and my symptoms. Looking back, however, I realized those items likely contained many harmful chemicals. In December 1989 I sought treatment for my cough and was given three trials of antibiotics but did not get relief. While symptoms of chemical sensitivity had been present for some time, I had no framework within which to relate them to chemical exposures. I lived with my symptoms and learned to tolerate them. After July 1990 I could no longer ignore my sensitivities to numerous chemicals, foods, and inhalants. My life became a matter of trying to survive in what had become a dangerous and toxic world. I wondered how many other people failed to recognize symptoms of chemical sensitivity and instead attributed their "dis-ease" to aging or other causes.

Even as I considered the origin of the strange sensitivities that my body had developed, I tried to carry on with my life. Attempting to lessen my symptoms, I reduced chemical exposures in my office at the child guidance center as much as possible. I removed an area rug bought five months earlier to brighten up that office, remembering how my coughing increased after I put it down. My coughing was so loud at times that it bothered people in the room next door. With the rug out of the way I coughed less. I also eliminated as many other potentially toxic items as I could. Despite these efforts I could not completely free myself of symptoms.

My anxiety level increased dramatically. I wanted to feel better, but no matter what I did I could not return to the way I used to feel. I controlled as much of my environment at home and at work as possible, but there was much that was not controllable. I recognized that pollution levels in the air outside my apartment had risen significantly in my twelve years there and worried this had contributed to my illness. I blamed myself for not noticing the change earlier and not moving to a place with healthier air. To lessen exposure to outdoor air pollution I kept my apartment's windows closed and used air filters. I stopped the three-times-a-week aerobic walking along the Charles River which I had done for years. More and more I felt the need to protect myself from the chemicals that were all around me.

Nothing in my past had prepared me for this crisis. For years I had valued my health and taken steps to maintain it. I had gone regularly for massage, acupuncture, psychotherapy, and chiropractic treatment. Daily practice of meditation had given me a sense of calm, but now my survival was threatened. In the past, meditation had served as a buffer against the stresses of the world. With the dramatic changes in my health there no longer was a buffer; there was only an ever-increasing sensitivity to my environment. No longer could I rely on my resources alone. I looked outside for help.

# CHAPTER TWO

# Seeking Outside Help

No matter what I did I could not make the constant muscle aching, dizziness, and confusion stop. As much as I preferred to depend on myself, I had to seek help from others. I had to visit my physician frequently and was grateful that she specialized in treating environmental illness. I learned many people with this disorder suffer for years without being given the correct diagnosis. They may consult several specialists, have numerous tests done, and be told nothing is wrong with them. They may be given medication that makes them worse. They may even be sent to a psychiatrist, because it is "all in their head." My physician worked with me to reduce my sensitivities.

I had undergone three rounds of intradermal allergy testing in June 1990 prior to the conference, first for inhalants like dust and molds, then for foods. During the testing sessions I experienced arm pain, dizziness, and confusion to a degree I never had before. In the third session my doctor decided the reason for my extreme reactions was sensitivity to phenol, a preservative used in the test substances. Based on the test results, I was given antigen drops to put under my tongue. One bottle was for dust, mites, and molds; a second was for eggs, corn, wheat, and milk; and a third was for glycerin, phenol, and alcohol. The idea was that taking the drops several times a week would lessen my reactivity.

While the testing indicated I already had sensitivities to inhalants, foods, and chemicals, it was the carpet exposure in July 1990 that pushed me over the edge. Before then my body could eventually clear any substance to which I was exposed, leading to the disappearance of symptoms. Thereafter the confusion, muscle aching, dizziness, and nausea never completely went away.

Within a few weeks the antigen drops made me feel worse and I stopped them. Although I had avoided medication in the past, I began regular use of an antihistamine for temporary relief. I also started an extensive regimen of nutritional supplements aimed at removing toxins and strengthening my immune system.

My heightened sensitivity affected all areas of my life. One example was dental care. A visit to the dentist was complicated by reactions to the chemicals in his office. When I told the hygienist about my problem, she replied she had never heard of such extreme reactions. I used a natural tooth powder instead of chemically laden toothpaste, switched to a natural-bristled toothbrush, and stopped using my mouthwash, which contained alcohol and other chemicals. The mouthwash killed germs but now also made me sick.

Frightened by the progression of my illness, I resorted to more extreme measures. Large doses of intravenous vitamin C cleared my head and relaxed my muscles, but the improvement was always only temporary. I wore a charcoal mask while driving and during acute exposures. When people made fun of me, I felt hurt and angry but could not be bothered for long. I was too busy trying to survive. A barrier cloth protected me from chemicals in the driver's seat of my car and reduced my back pain when I drove. I also considered changing my living situation.

Increasingly, I turned to Patty for support. She was the one person I knew who understood what I was going through. Not only did she have environmental illness, but it was also her job to work with people afflicted with it. We talked daily on the phone and saw each other often. She told me how her illness had developed and what she had done to cope with it.

She had begun to recognize something was wrong four years earlier while living in Florida. The headaches she had suffered with for years became progressively more frequent and, at times, incapacitating. She lived on over-the-counter pain relievers. Then the fatigue began. Fortunately, a yeast-free diet led to improvement.

The next year she moved to Brookline, Massachusetts, where she felt much worse, with more profound fatigue, headaches, ear pain, severe muscle and joint pain, and a constant cloudy feeling in her head. More and more of her time outside of work was spent sleeping and trying to deal with her pain. Just moving around became difficult. She found herself thinking this must be what it feels like to be suffering from radiation poisoning. She repeatedly saw images in her head of having survived a nuclear disaster.

From reading she had done Patty suspected her symptoms were related to food allergies and chronic candidiasis, a fungal infection. She searched long and hard for a doctor who would consider those possibilities as well as standard approaches. Finally, she found a holistically oriented physician whom she liked and who worked closely with her.

They connected the worsening of Patty's health with diesel fumes and pesticides she was constantly exposed to. The diesel fumes came from delivery trucks idling under the window of her Brookline apartment. Patty's landlord applied pesticides every three months to eliminate cockroaches. For days after the pesticides were sprayed, Patty felt them on her skin and tasted and smelled them. Her roommates did not appear affected. When Patty used cold water and baking soda to wipe down areas where the pesticides had been applied, as suggested by her doctor, she felt a little relief. Nonetheless, it became clear she needed to move in order to get better. Until she did so, she would feel miserable.

The house hunting was made particularly difficult by Patty's sensitivity to newsprint and car exhaust. Months of looking for a safe place led her to her Newburyport apartment. At first she managed the one-hour commute to her hospital job in Boston by carpooling with two other nurses. After the car pool fell apart, she drove one hour each way five or six days a week on her own. Trying to find a schedule she could manage, Patty decreased her hours at the hospital and began working part-time at the doctor's office where she had been a patient. That office also was an hour away. She explored getting a job closer to home, but the smaller suburban hospitals did not pay enough. She hoped cleaner air in Newburyport would more than offset high levels of pollution encountered by working in the city and commuting ten or more hours per week.

When Patty felt more exhausted and had trouble staying awake during her nightly drive home, her mother suggested she try an anti-depressant. Patty took a small dose of one under the guidance of her doctor, but felt great shame that she had to take such a medication to function. However, since it seemed to help, she continued on the antidepressant and tried to ignore feelings of being a failure.

Patty scheduled her jobs so that twice a month she had off three or four days in a row. On those days she slept, walked on the beach, soaked up the ocean air, and prayed she would regenerate herself enough to continue working. Often she felt exhausted and stayed in bed for much of her time off.

Efforts to make the apartment safe stretched Patty's finances to their limits. Her stove was one example. In her extensive search for a safe apartment she was unable to find a perfect one and compro-mised by accepting one with a gas stove. Since this was on the list of things to avoid, she paid to have the gas line to the stove shut off. She also had the apartment rewired for electric stove capacity and purchased a new electric stove. In that apartment she experienced a resultant decrease in muscle and joint pain, depression, ear pain, and brain fog, but within a month her symptoms slowly returned.

After weeks of feeling tired, depressed, dizzy, and nauseous, Patty suspected gas was still a problem. The plumber who had shut off the gas insisted her request to turn it off in the basement was unnecessary; he had capped it off in the apartment. Patty finally hired two other plumbers who did cap off the gas in the basement as she wanted. Then she felt much better. She had paid over a thou-sand dollars to have a stove she could safely use.

Although Patty spent several months and a great deal of money to create a safe environment, life in that apartment involved an ongoing struggle to avoid chemicals. Whenever people in the house next door used their clothes dryer, the antistatic agent gave off fumes that increased her weakness and joint pain. Patty learned that

Newburyport had community-wide spraying of Malathion which explained why she was unable to move some mornings during the summer. After a year there Patty acquired new downstairs neighbors who smoked and idled their truck under her living room windows for twenty minutes each morning. Cracked, leaky windows allowed exhaust fumes to fill her apartment, and her landlord's half-hearted attempts to repair them led to no improvement. Patty was too fearful to tell the neighbors the problems they were causing her and tolerated the daily exacerbation of her symptoms. She ran air filters while they warmed up their truck and then aired out her apartment once they left for the day.

Patty's relative stability was rudely shaken in March 1990 by a call from her landlord. She was stunned to learn that he wanted to live in her apartment. She had spent thousands of dollars to make it safe, and he was demanding she leave. He acknowledged the inconvenience he was causing and gave her three months notice.

Patty reacted to this announcement by going into a deep depression. Only after developing environmental illness myself would I understand the depth of her despair. She had done everything she could to protect herself from toxins, but one phone call from her landlord destroyed the limited security that had taken months to achieve. For weeks she avoided looking for a new apartment. Her memories of struggling to find a safe place two years earlier were still too overwhelming.

When she finally focused on moving, Patty did it quickly. She chose to live in Concord, a suburb west of Boston, where the air would be cleaner than in the city and the commute shorter than from Newburyport. Because she liked to cook, she placed an ad saying she wanted an apartment with a large kitchen. A professional couple responded with an unexpected offer of reduced rent for an apartment in their house if Patty cooked for them. The lower rent appealed to Patty because she wanted to further decrease her hours in the stressful coronary care unit.

Patty told the owner in detail about the importance of using less toxic materials in the renovations that needed to be done before she moved in. She also gave him the name of a handyman who used products having minimal toxins. While giving lip service to his willingness to meet her needs, the owner used his own carpenter and plumber.

Patty moved early in June while I was on a trip to Hawaii. Her mother flew in to help her pack and unpack. Patty later told me that from the moment she entered the apartment on the day she moved, she felt terrible. While previous trips there had not produced symptoms, on that day she knew something was horribly wrong. For the rest of her stay in Concord she had severe headaches, joint pain, intense spasms of her back muscles, and rock-hard shoulder muscles. An exhaustive search determined that the glues used to install a new kitchen sink were the cause of these latest symptoms. She learned such glues are extremely toxic and take a long time to outgas.

Patty again did everything she could to make this basement apartment livable. She tried to lessen fumes from the glue under the sink by having it sealed in a wooden box covered with a foil vapor barrier. She used fans to vent the toxic fumes out open windows but soon found mold growing in her bedroom closet. Patty then kept her windows closed. She ran air filters and bought an air conditioner to cool her apartment and a dehumidifier to dry it.

Despite her efforts Patty kept getting worse. By late July she was much sicker than when she moved. One day while walking outdoors to escape the glue, Patty smelled a strong, pungent odor that caused a chemical taste in her mouth, nausea, and muscle aching and spasms. She began to think that mold was at least as great a factor in the deterioration of her health as the plumber's glue. She talked with her doctor who told her Concord was in a basin and had significantly higher mold spore counts than Newburyport. Living there would mean constant mold exposure and mold-related symptoms.

This news alarmed Patty. Her new apartment exposed her to toxic chemicals and mold. She was increasingly incapacitated by new symptoms on top of the old ones. She had been too sick to cook for the landlord, so he wanted to raise her rent. With her savings and charge accounts exhausted by moving and trying to make the apartment safe Patty saw no way out of her predicament.

In early August Patty and I went to the beach seeking a respite from our problems. We hoped fresh ocean air would clear us of toxins, but even the ride there typified our battle with chemicals. Fifteen minutes into the hour-long trip we encountered a gigantic traffic jam. As we inched forward, exhaust fumes from outside accumulated in the car. I developed muscle spasms, confusion, and irritability. In a panic I screamed at Patty that we were supposed to be at the ocean feeling better; but instead we were stuck in a traffic jam, and I was being poisoned. My agitation grew as I feared these latest symptoms would be permanent. Although Patty reassured me the ocean air would clear my symptoms, I did not believe her. In the midst of this acute exposure my only point of reference was the near hysteria of the moment. I could not project ahead to the possibility of relief in the future.

We finally reached Gloucester and went to Wingaersheek Beach. My muscles ached. It was hard for me to walk. I was angry and felt nothing would help me. Patty cajoled me out of the car and down to the beach. We chose a place as far away as possible from others to avoid their cigarette smoke and perfume.

As we sat on the beach, layers of distress gradually left my body. First the muscle aching, then the irritability, then the confusion. Eventually, I looked around and noticed the beauty of the ocean, rocks, and blue sky. Patty felt better too. I felt so much better in the ocean air; I wanted never to leave. I wanted to feel well again, to end the suffering and uncertainty of endless reactions to chemicals, molds, and foods.

When dusk came, we prepared to leave and considered what to do next. We were each struggling with the seemingly insurmountable task of living with environmental illness in a toxic world. Patty suggested we move to a place together. At first her proposal startled me. For years I had enjoyed living alone, but environmental illness had totally changed my life, making it a constant battle for survival. I asked what she had in mind. She paused a moment and said we could help each other get better. I told her I would think about her idea.

The more I thought about Patty's suggestion the more sense it made. I worried that if I stayed where I was living, the air pollution would make me sicker. Tasks I had done quickly before now took much longer, like food preparation with the rotation diet. We already met nearly every day to assist each other with our individual crises. Perhaps together we would have more success than we were having alone.

I also had questions about her proposal. Although Patty usually had a warm, appealing personality, during reactions to various substances she had intense emotional outbursts. How would I cope with them? Would I be able to help her? How would we get along? What kind of relationship would we have? Where would we live? What would I do regarding work?

For several days the possibility of moving somewhere with Patty and my questions about it revolved in my mind until I became convinced the idea was a good one. It offered the potential for change and improvement. If living in the city had contributed to my illness, then moving might restore my health. Perhaps cleaner air in the country would help me to react less and to heal.

Without telling Patty, I looked at listings for apartments west of Boston. She was surprised when I showed her the ads during my next visit. She figured I had rejected her suggestion. When I told her I liked it, she was pleased and relieved. However, she felt the towns I had chosen were too close to metropolitan Boston and to major highways. We discussed which location and what kind of place would be best for us.

One important factor was the level of air pollution. We also wanted to be within a forty-minute commute of our jobs. For hours we drove along the roads of Boston's far western suburbs looking for towns with better air quality. After I read a newspaper article indicating air quality only improved beyond Route 495, we concentrated our search outside that beltway twenty-five miles from Boston.

I felt that living in a mountainous area was also important for our healing. The closest mountain west of Route 495 was Mt. Wachusett. Located in Princeton, it is the highest point in eastern Massachusetts and known for its scenic beauty. Commuting from Princeton would take over an hour. While we looked for rentals, we thought about how we could live there and keep our jobs.

Indoor air quality was another important factor. Needing to consider potential toxins when renting was new for me. In the past I had chosen apartments based on wanting to live there, not because of what I had to avoid. Now there was the pressure that if we did not choose wisely we could make ourselves worse.

Using Patty's past experience and consulting John Bower's book, *The Healthy House*, we came up with a list of requirements for a safe place to live. We wanted a three or four bedroom house that was older than twenty years with no recent construction and away from major roads. It should have hardwood floors, oil hot water heat, and a large kitchen with an electric stove. It should have many windows and receive plenty of sunlight. Any garage should be detached. There should be sufficient space around the house to protect it from neighbors' chemicals. Patty's two cats should be allowed. We wanted to pay no more than twelve hundred dollars per month and hoped to pay less.

With this list as a guide we looked at ads in local papers and called realtors. Most did not handle rentals. In other cases, as soon as we began to go over our list, they were not interested. When we looked at one place to learn what was available and at what price, its new paint and carpet made us sick. Another house was somewhat better, but its carpeting and paneling produced symptoms.

Grasping any potential lead, I called a realtor whose name was on a sign beside the road. After he heard I was a doctor, he listened to our requirements and said he had a condo that would meet our needs. We rushed to look at it. Despite his assurances about its safety, its obviously new construction brought on nausea and muscle aching. Thereafter, he did not return my calls.

Although our efforts to find a safe house in August failed, Patty gave her landlord notice. Under their three-month trial agreement she had to leave by mid-September. She felt so sick there she feared she might not even last that long. There was growing pressure to find a place right away.

Desperate for results we tried another approach. Since most of the rentals advertised were recently painted, we placed an ad aimed at reaching landlords earlier. It described our circumstances, asked them to contact us before renovating so that less toxic materials could be used, and offered to pay any additional costs. The ad was set to run the first Sunday in September.

At the end of August I meditated on our situation. We wanted to move to a house in the country near mountains. We had been unable to find a suitable place near Mt. Wachusett. I felt inspired to take a wider view of Massachusetts to see if there was another mountainous area that would offer more possibilities.

When I sat with a Massachusetts map in front of me, my attention was drawn to the southwest corner of the state. The name "Great Barrington" jumped out at me. I did not know the area, but remembered Jeff Rossman, a colleague who had relocated there a few years earlier. I obtained his phone number from directory assistance and called him immediately. Jeff was surprised to hear my voice. After we caught each other up on recent events, he told me in glowing terms about life in Great Barrington. Its strong points included the natural beauty of the Berkshires and numerous cultural events. He highly recommended living there.

I then called Patty and told her about my meditation and my conversation with Jeff. When I talked about the idea of moving to Great Barrington, she thought I was crazy. She asked how could we live in western Massachusetts and work in Boston? I replied that living there would be possible if I kept my apartment. I said I thought that we could stay in Watertown while working at our present jobs a few days a week. We would spend the rest of the time in the Berkshires, eventually living there full time.

Two days later we drove to Great Barrington. The 110-mile trip on the Massachusetts Turnpike took us through rolling hills and rocky terrain. Our ability to enjoy the scenery was limited by our reactions to exhaust fumes on the road. The fumes were always more intense when other cars accelerated up hills. Patricia was used to the increased muscle tension, nausea, and foggy-headedness that came with driving. I was not as tolerant of the nausea and joint and muscle pain that I experienced. The air conditioner pulled in air from outside so we tried to limit our exposure to the fumes by periodically turning the air conditioner off, running a portable air filter, and wearing charcoal masks. The trip turned out to be a delicate balance between too many exhaust fumes and too much heat.

After exiting the turnpike in Lee, we noticed a marked change. We were in the Berkshires. We took off our masks, opened the car windows, and breathed refreshing mountain air. Proceeding through picturesque Stockbridge, made famous by Norman Rockwell, we turned south on Route 7. A few miles later we stopped to rest at Monument Mountain on the outskirts of Great Barrington. After a brief walk, Patty sat in the driver's seat and rolled down the window to cool off the car. Within a minute she was behaving as if she were drunk. Her speech was slurred, and she flailed her arms around briefly before saying she could not move. It was several frightening moments before I discovered that the cover to her gas tank was missing and she was reacting to gasoline fumes. I took over driving and bought another gas cap at a nearby auto supply store.

Minutes later we were in the center of Great Barrington, a small town with historic homes and an inviting atmosphere. Its main street was lined with businesses, stores, and restaurants. Even in town we could feel the power of the mountains thrusting up around us. For me their presence was energizing and awe-inspiring. Patty felt them to be heavy and menacing. She found herself repeatedly thinking about the movie *The Shining*, a tale of murderous insanity set in the Rockies, based on the novel by Steven King. She chose not to tell me about these images for fear of spoiling our day with her negative thoughts. At the Chamber of Commerce we were greeted by cheerful ladies who eagerly gave us information about the area. On initial impression I thought Great Barrington seemed much friendlier than other places we had looked.

I called a number of realtors and finally spoke with one, who said she would be able to find a house that would meet our requirements. We agreed to meet her on Sunday, three days later. Patty and I liked the area so much we would consider moving there. The long commute would be a challenge, but having a safe and health-promoting house in the country would make the trip worthwhile.

When Sunday came, we wondered what would happen. What kind of response would there be to our ad for rentals in central Massachusetts? What would the realtor have to show us in Great Barrington?

Sunday morning the drive was more comfortable with much less traffic. Two and a half hours after leaving Watertown we were again in Great Barrington. The realtor showed us three places. The first two suggested she had not paid attention to our needs. One was carpeted throughout. The other was freshly painted. The third was a different story. To get there we drove to the outskirts of town and up a steep hill where the house sat nestled on the side of a gently rising mountain.

The large, two-story Cape's barn-red exterior contrasted sharply with its surroundings. Exploring the yard, we were impressed by the hills and mountains all around us and saw few other houses. Inside there were hardwood floors throughout. Heat was hot water by oil. The first floor included a good-sized kitchen with an electric stove, a large living room, three smaller rooms, and a large family room with windows on three sides. Upstairs were two large bedrooms. There were bathrooms on the first and second floors. The basement was large, wet, and filled with the owner's possessions. Beneath the kitchen was a garage.

We both felt a strong attraction to the house. We especially liked its location, the fact that it was a good distance from any neighbors, and its breathtaking views. It met most of our requirements, but we were very concerned about the water in the basement and the items stored there. We disliked the underhouse garage but could cope by not using it. We debated whether any of these difficulties should rule this house out.

Back at the realty office we discussed these issues. The realtor insisted the basement was wet only because the summer tenants had not properly ventilated it. She assured us the basement would be appropriately cleaned and dried out. Given our affinity for the house, the realtor's assurances, and Patty's urgent need to move, I wrote a check for the deposit. A meeting was arranged for the following Thursday with Jacob, the owner, to go over final details and to sign the lease.

That meeting went well. Jacob was a 45-year-old Yale geology professor. He cherished fond memories of this house where he had grown up and spoke proudly of how his grandfather had made the hand-hewn chestnut paneling in the kitchen and living room. When we described our reactions to chemicals, he listened attentively and agreed to use less toxic materials when repairs were made. He responded to questions about the wet basement by saying there were no leaks. He concurred with the realtor that any problem was caused by the summer tenants' keeping the basement closed up. He asked us to ventilate it well. We signed a year's lease and agreed to occupy the house on September fifteenth.

We then shifted from house hunting to getting ready to move. My sensitivities made this move more difficult than any I had done before. As packed boxes piled up in my apartment, I experienced fuzzy thinking, aching muscles, and a gluelike taste in my mouth, symptoms caused by the chemicals in cardboard. Together and separately Patty and I prepared to escape our reactions by moving to the country. Nothing, however, prepared us for the misadventures we would experience in the months ahead.

# CHAPTER THREE

# Escape to the Country

Patty and I prepared for the move with hope and anticipation. We looked forward to life in the country with clean, fresh air and improved health. At the same time we worried about how the arrangement would work out. We recognized the absurdity of moving to a house two-and-a-half hours away from our jobs but had been unable to find a suitable place closer. Interestingly, we did receive several responses to our ad for the Mt. Wachusett area, but only after the lease for the house in Great Barrington had been signed.

With little more than a week to go I helped Patty pack the belongings her mother had helped her unpack just three months earlier. I also packed most of my things. There were boxes and boxes of books covering a wide range of topics. The majority were about healing, science, and yoga. I decided to leave only the basic necessities we would need in my apartment during our two-and-a-half days a week in the Boston area.

Patty's friend Jim agreed to help us move. Early Friday morning I went with him to pick up a twenty-six-foot U-Haul truck, which he drove back to Watertown. He was surprised by how much I had packed. Jim and his friend Dan spent four hours filling the truck and then stopped to have room for Patty's possessions. At the time I felt irritated that not all my things made it onto the truck. Fifteen months later I would be grateful not everything I owned had gone to Great Barrington.

We drove to Patty's apartment; and when we started loading her things, it soon became apparent the truck was not big enough.

While Jim and Dan continued loading, Patty and I went to get a second truck. We were able to rent a fourteen-footer. When we returned, the first truck was filled, and they were ready to start on the second. By seven o'clock the loading was done, and we were exhausted. Already the move was more than we had planned for.

Early Saturday morning our caravan headed west on the Turnpike. I led in my station wagon loaded with items too fragile to pack with anything else. Jim drove the twenty-six-foot truck. Patty had moved so many times she was by now an experienced truck driver and took the wheel of the fourteen-footer. Dan followed in his car. As I drove west, I felt I was leaving my past behind and had a sense of optimism about the new beginning which lay ahead, about our new life in the mountains. I hoped this move would allow me to regain my health. If being well again meant moving to the westernmost end of Massachusetts, I was willing to do that. For the present, my symptoms were worse as a result of the chemical exposures involved in packing and moving.

Slowed by the trucks our trip to Great Barrington took longer than usual. Upon our arrival Dan and Jim strolled around the yard, enjoying the warm sunshine and refreshing southerly breezes of the late summer day, and admiring the expansive views of the surrounding mountains. After their break they rapidly unloaded the trucks so that they could be back in Boston that evening. When they left at five o'clock, Patty and I were alone in our new home.

The house, which had been nearly empty when we first looked at it, was now filled with our boxes and furniture. We maneuvered our way around them to examine its condition. Upstairs the east bedroom's slanted ceiling had a new, three-inch-wide dent. The landlord had left many more things than expected, including a dresser with drawers that reeked of perfume. With improved ventilation the basement was dry, but we were appalled to find it still filled with the landlord's belongings, paint supplies, and construction materials.

We both were excited about how much space the house had to offer and began considering how to allocate it. I thought about using one of the small first-floor rooms as my bedroom but noticed an unpleasant odor which we could not identify. We would spend months trying to discover its source. If I used the upstairs west bedroom, I would want to paint over its ugly pink trim. I needed rooms for an office and a library; Patty wanted an exercise room. She had already appropriated the second-floor east bedroom because of its view south to Mt. Everett. We could share it until I decided where my bedroom would be. When Patty told me she disliked having separate bedrooms, I explained that my yoga teacher recommended each person have his or her own space and that sleep was a time to renew energies. Patty did not understand, yet felt she had no choice but to agree.

After clearing Patty's bedroom of boxes, we slept soundly, breathing in the country air. I awakened the next morning to find a deer on the lawn and roused Patty so that she could see it too. We interpreted the deer's presence as an indication we had found a place that would bring us the healing we were looking for. We had escaped the city!

We began the day by stretching and meditating outside on the grass. The setting was so beautiful. It reminded me of magnificent retreats where I had studied yoga in California, Hawaii, and Vermont.

Later in the morning I called Jacob and asked what he wanted done with the things he had left. He said to store them in the basement. I also informed him of the new dent in the ceiling. He said he would have his handyman, Harold, repair the dent along with the other items we had discussed earlier. When I reminded him of his agreement to use nontoxic products in any repairs, he again expressed willingness to do so.

On Monday we woke early and prepared for our two-and-a-half-hour commute to Boston. We wanted to establish a new rhythm of relaxation and healing in the country and working in the city. It never turned out as we had hoped, but we did have the flexibility in our work schedules to try. Patty changed her hours at the doctors' office and began working late Monday morning. I started Monday afternoon. We planned to work Monday through Wednesday and return to Great Barrington Wednesday night or Thursday morning.

My chemical sensitivities required me to make many changes at my job. While a sportscoat had been standard attire for me, I no longer could wear one. The linings of all my sportcoats now made me sick. Instead, I wore a shirt and tie and added a sweater when it was colder. To protect myself from chemicals and particulate matter in the air I used a large air filter. I put a barrier cloth over my vinyl covered office chair to minimize the muscle spasms and muscle pain I had when I sat in it.

My superiors put up with these changes but expressed concern about the effects my walking into the clinic with a brown box and a white sheet would have on others. I agreed to send a memo to other clinicians and staff informing them of my health problem and explaining my new equipment. I gave the memo a humorous tone, but beneath the humor was a deep sense of fear, frustration, and sadness that I had to resort to such measures to be able to keep working.

When Patty and I returned to Great Barrington, we both experienced a strong feeling of déjà vu each time we walked up the front steps and stood on the porch. We assumed this was a good sign, that it meant we had found the right place. Over the next two weekends we emptied most of the boxes for the kitchen. The rest of the boxes we stored out of the way in the family room. Patty and I were aware of some symptoms in the house but felt they must be related to the boxes.

By the third week we were certain something in the kitchen was causing fatigue and muscle spasms. We smelled the floor, the cabinets, and the walls and discovered the wooden walls were covered with layers of polish. Using a low toxicity cleaner called "Super Clean" and water, we removed it. We had to be careful not to use too much Super Clean. Otherwise we reacted to it too. After we cleaned and rinsed the walls four times, our latest symptoms went away.

As more cold weather occurred, the house was closed up more and we again experienced more brain fog, confusion, muscle tightness, fatigue, and nausea. We searched for toxins in the house which might be causing these problems. During a trip to the basement a shelving unit loaded with cans of paint thinner, gasoline, turpentine, and chemicals caught Patty's eye. She observed that these substances were all potential sources of our symptoms. To eliminate them I bought three large aluminum trash cans, put them outside, filled them with the offending agents, and sealed them with foil tape. Once those chemicals were removed, the air in the basement lightened; and we had fewer symptoms.

The three small rooms on the first floor still did not feel right to me. While I was considering choosing one of them for my bedroom, I was reluctant to do so given the nausea, muscle aching, and spaciness I felt there. To eliminate any mold or chemicals in those rooms we spent hours washing them from floor to ceiling. Five weeks after we moved in, the rooms were cleaner than they had been in years, but my discomfort persisted. I suspected something else in the basement was causing the problem. Since experts in environmental medicine recommend your bedroom be the place where you have least toxic exposures, I decided to use the west bedroom on the second floor.

We not only found many toxins that needed to be eliminated but inadvertently created new problems for ourselves. When Harold came to make some repairs, I gave him a special joint compound that was supposed to be safe for people with chemical sensitivities. He used it to fill the dent in Patty's bedroom ceiling. After he was done, we both became sick in that room with drowsiness, dizziness, and incoordination.

I called the company where I bought the joint compound and asked their advice. They said it would be okay once it dried. We tried using heaters to dry the joint compound, but the heat only made things worse. In addition, the joint compound shrank so that it no longer filled the dent. We then used fans to dry it. After several days the fumes were less. Meanwhile, we slept with the bedroom windows wide open and suffered. Eventually, we covered the dent with a vapor barrier called "denny foil" and told Harold not to work on it any more.

I was discovering how much chemical sensitivities could complicate my life. I had to be extremely careful about whatever I did. If I made a mistake, I could feel sicker than I did already and that feeling could last for hours or days.

Even with this growing awareness, I still tried to function as if my life were normal. In October I noticed rust above the rear wheels of my car and decided to have it repaired before the rust spread. I took my car to the bodyshop in Pittsfield which had given the lowest estimate, told them about my sensitivities, and emphasized the importance of not painting inside the car. When I picked my car up, I promptly developed nausea and muscle spasms. I looked where they had painted and was shocked to find that in repairing the rust they had painted inside the rear door as well as the outside of the car. The paint fumes were making me sick and probably were now on the upholstery. I was frightened about making the thirty-minute drive back to Great Barrington to say nothing about the long trip to Boston.

I learned that the paints used in autobody work were extremely toxic for me. There was no easy or quick way to remedy the situation. The paint fumes would dissipate eventually, but it was impossible to say how long that would take. As soon as I arrived back at our home, which we now called the Red House, I opened the car doors and tried to correct the problem. I put two heaters on folding chairs and began heating the newly painted areas. I alternated hours of heating with hours of ventilating by fans but without success. It was weeks before I could try using my car again and months before I would feel all right in it. Until then, Patty and I shared her car.

In mid-October we had dinner with my friend Jeff Rossman and his wife at a local restaurant that served brown rice. We arranged to go on the rice day of our rotation diet. I told Jeff about our illness and asked that they not use any scented, personal care products. He was surprised by my request but agreed to comply. We enjoyed our evening with them. It was refreshing to hear how much they liked the Berkshires and about cultural events they had attended. We did not realize that our sensitivities would worsen to such an extent that we would never enjoy any of those cultural offerings during our nineteen months there. It would be a long time before we tried socializing again.

Patty was having symptoms not only in Great Barrington but also in Watertown. She felt that the five-year-old mattress in my apartment caused her to wake up in the morning with joint pain, muscle aching, and a puffy face. She insisted I buy a cotton futon, which she said experts in environmental illness recommended over a foam mattress, because the former had fewer chemicals. When she lived in Newburyport, Patty had purchased a futon to replace the foam mattress she had recently acquired. With that change, her joint pain and puffy morning face had gone away.

Eager to do what I could to lessen our exposure to toxins, I agreed to buy a futon. Our schedules were so full, it was difficult even to find time to shop for one. A couple of weeks later we managed to race to a store in Cambridge just before closing time. After selecting a futon, we were ready to take it home but were frustrated to learn they did not have one in stock at the store. We would have to pick it up at their warehouse during business hours.

The next week we squeezed a trip to the warehouse into our hectic schedules. Shortly after the futon was loaded into the car, my tension level started to climb. I smelled chemicals and my muscles became taut all over. I asked Patty if she noticed the smell. She replied her futon had an odor at first but was fine after she aired it out and put a barrier cloth cover on it.

Patty did not react to the futon right away, but by the time we reached Watertown she was feeling tired and achy too. We carried the futon up the stairs and put it in the back room to air out. Although we kept that room's windows open, the strong chemical smell spread throughout the apartment. The futon's fumes caused us to have flulike symptoms and mental cloudiness. In an effort to contain the fumes, I covered the door between the kitchen and the back room with denny foil. The denny foil helped some, but our goal was to be able to sleep on the futon.

Patty's friend Sherry told us she had used ozone to eliminate chemicals on her things. We learned ozone is a triatomic form of oxygen which is both toxic and able to neutralize chemicals. Sherry loaned us her ozone machine to treat the futon. We prepared the back room, turned the machine on, and closed the door. At first we stayed in the apartment while the ozone machine was running, but our muscles became so weak we could barely move. We left before becoming completely immobilized. When we returned three hours later, we turned the machine off and aired the room out. Even after ozoning, the futon had a strong smell which neither of us could stand.

We wondered why this futon was so different from the one Patty bought only two years earlier. When I called the store where we purchased it, they said new federal regulations required a significant increase in the amount of fire retardant used. Patty and I were feeling the effects of this change. Eventually, after several more tries at ozoning, we gave up and put the futon in the basement.

The frustrations of life with environmental illness continued to mount. Repeatedly I encountered situations where chemicals made me sick. Trying to correct the problem often made things worse or life more complicated. Patty had resigned herself to always being chemically sensitive and to having persistent symptoms since her doctor had told her this would be the case. I remembered research by psychologist Martin Seligman on learned helplessness. When he placed dogs in experimental conditions where they had no control, they learned to give up. I was not ready to give up but recognized that having environmental illness definitely increased my feelings of helplessness.

In October we discovered another threat at the Red House. We noticed mysterious, tiny, black curlycues on the bed where Patty's cats had been. At the same time, I was bothered by repeated insect bites on the tops of my feet and the lower part of my legs. Detective work led us to conclude we had a flea infestation. The fleas especially liked biting me, which was compounded by the danger that they would further overstimulate my immune system.

Remembering the large number of flea bites I suffered during my trip to Hawaii that May, I became convinced they had been one of the factors setting me up for immune-system overload.

Eradicating the fleas became a top priority. We took Patty's cats to a local vet who confirmed the diagnosis and who said it would be easy to eliminate the fleas. He recommended washing the cats and setting a few flea bombs. Patty and I stared at each other in horror; the vet had no idea how dangerous those bombs would be for us with our heightened sensitivities. When Patty tried using a pyrethrum-based spray, one of the supposedly more benign products, three rooms away from me, I instantly developed extreme weakness and neuromuscular incoordination. Unable to swallow or speak, I moaned loudly to get her attention. She immediately stopped spraying, opened the windows, and cleaned up the area where she had been working. I was grateful to be able to swallow again.

I felt trapped between the flea bites, which overstimulated my immune system, leading to greater sensitivity, and products to kill the fleas which made me dangerously sick. We sought alternative solutions through the BioIntegral Resource Council in California. They suggested starting with frequent shampooing of the cats, using a flea comb, and regular vacuuming. We implemented these measures, but the fleas persisted. As we understood more about the life cycle of the fleas and how hardy their eggs could be, we realized it would be a challenge to find products that would kill both adult fleas and flea eggs and still be safe for us. Frequent vacuuming, combing, and cat baths became part of the routine in Great Barrington while we looked for a solution.

Clearly, I now had more problems than when I moved to the Red House. In support of my desire to heal myself, I consulted a local homeopathic physician who treated people with immune dysfunction. When I arrived at his office, I checked in with the receptionist and then sat in the waiting room. My attention was drawn to the shiny floor. Noticing tightness in the muscles of my back, arms, and legs and constriction in my chest, I charged over to the receptionist and demanded to know what had been done to the floor. She replied they had polyurethaned it the week before. I was enraged that I was being assaulted by such a strong toxin in the doctor's office where I had gone for help. I said I could not stay there. She offered to let me wait in another room that had not been polyurethaned.

When the doctor came to speak with me, he apologized for the difficulty I was having. I expressed my outrage that, given the kind of patients he treated, he had used polyurethane on the floor. He offered a lame excuse but appeared to have no concept of the toxic effects of chemicals. We met in his office with the windows wide open. When the appointment was over, I was glad to leave. The outcome of my visit was that he prescribed two homeopathic remedies that I could not tolerate. When I tried them, I became dizzy and nauseous in spite of adjustments in the dose.

When I mentioned my problems with the standard remedies to a friend in New Mexico, she told me about a man named Jon Monroe who did electronic homeopathy. I called to find out what he had to offer. Combining his background in electronics and biology, Jon had invented a device that he said read the electronic pattern of a substance placed in it and then created an inverse pattern to be transmitted to a remedy. He recommended we start with an autodetox remedy that would support our bodies' efforts to eliminate toxins. As requested, Patty and I each sent him Kleenex with a drop of urine on it. In a few days we received our remedies, which we were able to take without any adverse reactions.

In the midst of our ongoing difficulties settling into Great Barrington, we had to find ways to pay for this new lifestyle. Both Patty and I had expected to feel better in the country and assumed we would be able to work more hours. Thus far, moving in had been a full-time job.

The idea of finding additional work raised the question of what kind of place would be safe for us. I looked for a job with flexibility as to how long I would have to spend inside at any one time and arranged to do one day of psychiatric consultations a week in either

Pittsfield or Auburn. Pittsfield was half an hour's drive north of Great Barrington. Auburn was forty-five minutes west of Watertown on the way to Great Barrington. The offices that were available had older carpet and some old particle-board-type furnishings. I performed the consultations with filtered air blowing on my face and went outside for fresh air between appointments.

Patty was also concerned about where she would work. She no longer wanted to be involved with the kind of high-stress, high-tech nursing she had done in critical care for years. In November she found a small hospital in Great Barrington where the pace in the intensive care unit was more to her liking. Fortunately, the chemical exposures in that unit were relatively low. She agreed to work there on a per diem basis two weekends a month beginning in January 1991.

By late November our schedules were packed. We made the long commute to Boston on Monday mornings and worked there from Monday through Wednesday. I worked alternate Thursdays in Auburn. On those days, Patty went grocery shopping and prepared for the trip back to the Red House. My days in Great Barrington were filled with cleaning the house, doing laundry, and dictating reports for my new job. Patty shopped for groceries, cooked all our meals, washed lots of dishes, and did flea control. Alternate Saturdays I worked in Pittsfield. The rest of the time we focused on trying to solve the problems, which continued to emerge in connection with our chemical sensitivities.

Our return to the Red House was often emotionally draining. Many times, after a few minutes in the kitchen, Patty would begin sobbing and then complained she had no energy, that she could not stand up. This behavior was a marked and sudden change, and we tried to find a cause for it. Was it from physical exhaustion, from depression, or from a chemical exposure in the house? The change was so abrupt we felt it must be caused by something in the house. It would be a long time before we had a clearer picture of what was behind this collapsing in the kitchen.

By mid-November we began preparing for winter. When the

heat was turned on, dust on the radiators sent me into fits of cough-ing. I spent one weekend cleaning them. All the dirt I found sug-gested it had not been done in years. Afterward I coughed less with the heat on.

We needed coverings for the windows to prevent heat loss to the outside. The curtains we found in stores had too many chemicals. As an alternative we bought cotton sheets to use as curtains. We washed them numerous times to remove their chemicals but with-out success. We then ozoned the sheets but that did not work either. As a last resort we put denny foil over the windows. This solution aggravated Patty. She said it felt like we were living in a dungeon. I did not like it either, but at least the foiled windows kept heat in and did not make us sick.

Finding I no longer could wear my winter coats, which were made of nylon and polyester, I shopped for a down parka that had a cotton shell and cotton lining. When I finally found one, it need-ed to be washed fifteen times before I could tolerate wearing it. In general I had not been able to wear new clothes in over six months. Despite washing pants, shirts, or underwear more than twenty times they still bothered me.

Even with our many difficulties I still wanted the Red House to work out. I contracted with Harold to paint the upstairs west bed-room. He used good-quality latex paint mixed with baking soda, a suggestion Patty had learned was supposed to create outgassing of harmful chemicals in paint. After Harold was done, we aired the room out repeatedly. Unfortunately, we developed nausea and mus-cle cramping whenever we entered it. I put denny foil over its door to seal the fumes off from the rest of the house and aired the room out daily. When I checked with an expert on safe products, she told me baking soda in paint removes odors but does not neutralize harmful chemicals. Reactions to the paint would persist.

This discouraging failure on the paint front was quickly over-shadowed by the need to address other problems. By early December, we had completed research on the best way to approach the fleas. Any successful intervention had to attack both adult fleas and the flea eggs. We learned diatomaceous earth is effective at killing adult fleas by poking holes in their skeletons. We found a product that combined diatomaceous earth with pyrethrums, insecticides derived from chrysanthemums. The pyrethrums would prevent the flea larvae from becoming sexually active adults. In order to eradicate the fleas the diatomaceous earth had to be left down for ten days.

We tested how the diatomaceous earth affected each of us. It irritated my lungs tremendously, causing paroxysms of coughing. Patty experienced intense muscle aching, but felt she could cope with it.

Early on the morning of December tenth, we implemented the flea attack plan. Patty covered as much of herself as she could with her shower cap, charcoal mask, rain suit, socks, and sneakers. Looking like someone ready to enter a decontamination chamber, she spread diatomaceous earth on all the floors and other surfaces where the cats went. She threatened to kill me when I tried to take a picture of her. As soon as the task was completed, she took off the protective gear and we drove to Boston.

I avoided the diatomaceous earth by staying in Watertown for the next ten days. When Patty returned to the Red House that Thursday, she found the interior to be like a battle zone. A coating of dust covered everything. Dead bodies of fleas, mature and immature adults, were scattered everywhere. She stayed for a few days to be with her cats and then drove back to Watertown. The next Thursday, December twentieth, she returned to the Red House to vacuum the dust and the dead fleas.

I arrived the following morning and was relieved to learn the fleas were gone. Even though Patty had vacuumed everywhere, enough diatomaceous earth remained to trigger my coughing. We had to wash all the surfaces in the house with damp cloths before I could breathe comfortably again. This activity reminded Patty of wiping down her Brookline apartment for pesticides, only this job was much bigger. She thought of how her life had become nothing more than a series of endless tasks to make her environment safe and wondered if it would ever change.

As 1990 ended, Patty and I looked forward to 1991. We hoped that the most difficult times were behind us. Eradicating the fleas was a major accomplishment. We had also overcome many other obstacles over the last three-and-a-half months and survived. It was time for things to start improving. We spent the last week of the year at the Red House. It was a chance to enjoy the natural beauty that surrounded us. Feeling some increased energy from using the autodetox remedy, we looked forward to 1991 as a beginning of renewed health.

# CHAPTER FOUR

# There Is No Escape

By January 1991 Patty and I had been through more than enough. We wanted to leave the moving and the chemical reactions behind us. It was a new year and we wanted to go forward with our lives. We tried to convince ourselves things would work out. Even if I could not yet use my recently painted bedroom, we could manage that. Eventually, it would be possible to air out the room sufficiently so that I would be able to sleep there. The strain of the long-distance commuting could be managed once we made the house safe. We hoped to escape the ongoing trauma of environmental illness but would soon realize how futile our hopes were.

Patty's efforts to resume her life included her new job in Great Barrington and learning how to reclaim her "name." She started working alternate weekends on the day shift in the critical care unit at Fairview Hospital where she introduced herself as "Patricia." "Patricia" was her given name, but growing up she had been called "Patty." She used the name Patty because that was what people called her. I had talked with her about the importance of the name we use—our name embodies our sense of our self and carries energy to us when people speak it. When she meditated on her names, she decided that "Patty" made her feel like a child and that "Patricia" was stronger and more in harmony with her true sense of herself.

I encouraged Patricia to use the name she felt most strengthened by. Ten years earlier I experienced the healing effects of the name when aligned with one's inner being. I studied with sound healers, Sarah Benson and Molly Scott, who led an exercise called the "Song

55

of the Soul." In the exercise, one person stands in the center of a circle while others surrounding him chant his name. When I stood in the center and "Robert" was chanted, I noticed feelings of deep relaxation, energization, and expansion. Thereafter I made a concerted effort to be called "Robert" instead of "Bob," which is the norm in our culture. I discovered how difficult it was for people to change what they called me regardless of my request that they do so.

Patricia was surprised by how she reacted when people called her by her new name. When hospital staff called to "Patricia," she assumed they were talking to someone else. Upon realizing they were addressing her, she wondered why they were so formal until she remembered that was how she had introduced herself. It took many months for her to identify herself as Patricia.

In January I tried to resume my study of *qi gong* (pronounced chee gong), a form of exercise and movement practiced widely in China for health. I last studied it in May 1990 during two weeks at a Taoist monastery in Hawaii shortly before I became sick. I called Claude Lawrence, who had advertised qi gong classes in Lenox and asked about the content of the class and possible chemical exposures. I wanted to know whether the classroom had been recently renovated and whether any students wore scented personal care products. Satisfied by Claude's answers, I decided to observe a class.

Patricia deeply resented the prospect of my going. Prior to her developing environmental illness, aerobic exercise had been essential to maintaining her physical and emotional well-being. When Patricia's sensitivities prohibited her from taking exercise classes in several different settings, she purchased an exercise bicycle, a new television, and a VCR so that she could work out at home. She did that for a while, but her two moves within four months in 1990 had caused so much disruption and her life was so complicated and demanding that now she no longer had time to exercise. She thought of my plans to study qi gong while she washed yet another pile of dishes and tried to ignore her anger.

In mid-January I went to my first class at the Community

Center in Lenox. I met Claude Lawrence, whose presence embodied fluid movement and grounding. To my relief none of the other three students wore scents that bothered me. I agreed to register for the class with the understanding I would need to make adjustments should problems with chemicals arise. Aiming to prevent exposures, I asked the others to continue to be free of strong-smelling personal-care products. I attended three classes before my life collapsed in February.

During January, Harold, who worked part-time as a handyman and full-time doing maintenance for a local school, began completing the repairs at the Red House which he had begun in the fall. Although Harold seemed well-intentioned, we had a difficult time when he came to the house. His aftershave had such a potent smell that it aggravated our symptoms. Choosing to avoid imposing our limitations on him, we did not tell him the aftershave made us sick; but we always felt relieved when he left. We looked forward to the day when all the repairs would be done so that we would no longer have to smell his cologne.

One major project remained: painting the first floor bathroom. An outside wall and the adjacent ceiling had water damage and a moldy smell, which forced us to keep the bathroom door closed. In late January, I talked with Harold by phone about his plans. He wanted to scrape off the old paint and then apply primer, followed by two coats of paint. I told him we wanted to use paint products that were safe for chemically sensitive people. After I hung up the phone, I talked with Patricia about the conversation. She was appalled that I had agreed to his plan and insisted I tell him to hold off until spring when we could adequately ventilate the room. I called Harold back and left a message on his answering machine to that effect. Monday morning we drove to Boston confident the bathroom project was "on hold."

When we returned to the Red House three days later, our lives were totally blown apart. Upon entering the front door, Patricia and I were overcome by dizziness and nausea. We needed to identify what was wrong. Going into the first-floor bathroom revealed the answer—our nausea and dizziness intensified. We were assaulted by a potent odor that neither of us recognized. There was fresh paint on the ceiling and walls; despite my message Harold had worked on the bathroom. Panic and rage gripped me. What had he done? What could we do to correct this new and most distressing problem?

Right away, I opened the window to try to air out the bathroom. I then called Harold and demanded to know what had transpired. He said he had applied shellac and primer. I pressed him to find out why he ignored my message on his answering machine. He claimed he never received it. When I asked why not, he replied that perhaps the machine was not working. I found this response hard to believe. Earlier on the day I called, the machine worked fine. I suspected Harold, having had enough of modifying his actions for our needs, went ahead with the bathroom the way he wanted. He planned to use regular paint color-coordinated with the rest of the bathroom. He would add baking soda to minimize toxic fumes. He said he had not been paid for what he had done at the Red House since the fall and would receive payment only when all the work was completed. I repeated how angry I was and told him Patricia and I would discuss what we wanted done about the bathroom.

Patricia and I tried to figure out what to do, but by then our thinking was quite muddled. I called a company specializing in products for chemically sensitive individuals and described the situation. They said shellac posed a serious hazard for anyone with sensitivities. Its effects could be both debilitating and long-lasting. Different interventions could be tried to eliminate shellac, but each had limitations. The easiest remedy was to air the room out. Since it was mid-winter, airing would not be as effective as it would be in the summer. We could try to mechanically remove the shellac, but that might ruin the walls. We could try sealing the shellac with paint or a sealant. Then we would have to cope with any reactions to that substance. Or we could try to neutralize the shellac by ozoning.

Fumes from the bathroom made us feel sick throughout the house. All my muscles were in spasms. I noticed the tightness especially in my arms and legs. Sometimes my legs weakened suddenly and I caught myself falling forward. Although it was February and the temperature outside was in the teens, we now kept all the windows open while we were in the house. Even with these measures, we could only stay there for two days—we had to leave to avoid becoming even sicker. Before we left, I called Harold and told him he might as well try painting over the shellac. We hoped the paint would seal the shellac fumes, and we would be able to tolerate being in the house.

We delayed our next return to the Red House by two days. The trip from Boston to Great Barrington was no longer an escape from the toxins of the city to the safety of the country but a return to confront shellac fumes, primer, and now paint, used to try to seal the other two. As soon as we entered the house, my dizziness and muscle aching again increased. Since the temperature inside was below sixty-five degrees, I turned the thermostat up. Shortly after the heat came on, my dizziness and muscle aching worsened further and I developed abdominal cramping. Patricia had similar symptoms.

When we looked for the cause of these symptoms, we discovered an open can of paint on the radiator in the downstairs bathroom. After the heat came on, the radiator warmed the can and sent paint fumes into the air and through the house. Right away I sealed the can and took it outside. I had spoken extensively with Harold about our chemical sensitivities and the importance of minimizing exposures to chemicals. He had listened and nodded his head as if he understood. Obviously he had not. We could hardly believe this chain of events.

We had hoped sealing the shellac with paint would lessen our symptoms, but instead we felt worse. Patricia's bedroom had been the room where we felt best. Now we had symptoms there too. We debated whether staying overnight was safe. We tried sleeping with the windows wide open, but awakened feeling very achy with sore joints and extreme fatigue. We concluded we could not sleep in the house again until there was significant reduction of the toxins in the bathroom.

Slowly, the reality of this latest complication began to sink in. We now faced the challenge of trying to make the Red House safe while not being able to stay there. To complicate matters, the place where we could stay was two-and-a-half hours away. We felt shell-shocked as we tried to figure out what to do.

Patricia had read of a technique called "bake-out," which is used to eliminate chemicals in new buildings. In a bake-out, the building is closed up and the heat is set on high. The high heat increases chemical outgassing and reduces the overall chemical level. Nancy Sokol Green, author of *Poisoning Our Children: Surviving in a Toxic World*, writes that a bake-out can increase outgassing by 400 percent and reduce chemicals by 25 percent. (p. 99) After a bake-out, it is important to air the building out well before reentering it.

Our trips to Great Barrington now were basically to try to make the house habitable again and to go to the jobs we had taken to pay for this lifestyle that no longer worked. We brought an electric, oil-filled, radiant heater to heat the first-floor bathroom and left it on while we were gone. When we returned, I opened windows to air the house out and sat in my car while the bake-out fumes dissipated. When I went into the house, my nausea, dizziness, muscle aching, abdominal cramping, and mental confusion still worsened. I even had difficulty finding the words I wanted to say. Often when I spoke, the wrong word came out of my mouth.

My mind, which had been one of my greatest assets, no longer worked for me. It had enabled me to graduate first in my high school class, obtain an undergraduate degree from Yale with honors, and then complete medical school at the University of Pennsylvania. Previously, I might have been frightened by this deterioration in mental functioning, but now I just felt overwhelmed and numbed by what I was going through. We were so caught up in survival tasks that occupied every minute of every hour that we were unable to comprehend fully what was happening.

We used whatever interventions we could think of to cope with the effects of these latest exposures. We resumed weekly treatments with our acupuncturist, Kiiko Matsumoto, a brilliant clinician and internationally known teacher. Those treatments brought temporary relief of muscle spasms and brain fog for which we were both grateful. We continued using the autodetox remedy. While it helped, our bodies now had much more to detoxify. We took more magnesium orally to lessen muscle spasms. Once again we resorted to intravenous vitamin C. We learned that a baking soda soak in the bathtub can help detoxify the body, so we took soaks in Watertown as often as we could. The soaks led to some welcome muscle relaxation and clearer thinking.

By the end of February, Patricia and I were in a panic. Three weeks had gone by since Harold shellacked the bathroom. We had baked it out repeatedly to no avail. Any time inside the Red House was spent huddled in our winter coats with the windows wide open.

The emergence of new symptoms amplified our emotions even more. Patricia complained of "butt pinching," which radiated down the back of her right leg. One day as she walked across the living room, the pain suddenly became so severe that she fell to the floor in tears. My own fears about the cause of her pain and its implications filled my head. I felt totally helpless and cried too as I remembered my mother's debilitating, chronic back pain. The house that was supposed to help us heal had become an ongoing, living nightmare.

Out of growing desperation, I called our landlord, Jacob, to inform him of our latest troubles. I hoped he might have suggestions, but he was away on business. I spoke instead with his wife Sarah. She was surprised to hear of our reactions to the work in the bathroom and was most upset by my report of Patricia's severe sciatic pain and difficulty walking. I said we would have to take stronger measures if we were to make the house livable for us. She offered no advice but agreed to our using denny foil to seal the bathroom off from the rest of the house and to ozoning. When I mentioned Harold's belief that he would not be paid for work done thus far until the entire repair list was completed, she responded that of course her husband would pay him for finished work if there were jobs that needed to wait until warmer weather.

Perhaps if Harold had known he would be paid, he might have delayed painting the bathroom until spring. Now Patricia and I had to live with the consequences of his actions. We stayed in the Red House a few more hours that Saturday. Shiatsu massage on Patricia's back and legs gave some relief. Otherwise she rested or limped around. We both had constant, painful, muscle spasms in our feet. I used two rolls of denny foil to seal the first-floor bathroom off from the rest of the house as much as possible. I put a double layer of denny foil over the bathroom door and covered all the walls on the outside of the bathroom. I put a double layer of denny foil on the floor of the upstairs bathroom, which was directly over the downstairs one. Covering these surfaces seemed to help. When the denny foil ran out, we drove back to Watertown to get away from the chemicals in the Red House.

Patricia saw her chiropractor on Monday and was relieved to learn she did not have an injury to her lower back. The chiropractor said she had extreme muscle spasm that was causing the pain in her buttocks and leg. He advised stretching exercises and avoiding shellac.

Until then our symptoms had been familiar to us. The cramping abdominal pain, the muscle spasms in our feet, and Patricia's sciatic pain were frightening new developments. I also began having muscle spasms in my hands, especially when holding something made of plastic, and had to start wearing cotton gloves while driving to protect myself from the vinyl of the steering wheel. I also switched from the plastic ballpoint pens I had been using to metal writing pens.

The Watertown apartment was now our "safe" place; but, as a result of our exposure to paint and shellac at the Red House, we began also having symptoms in the Watertown kitchen and bathroom. My landlord had painted those rooms the previous June at my request. While I had not reacted to the paint before, I now began having symptoms like those I was having in Great Barrington, including muscle aching, cramping abdominal pain, fatigue, nausea, and confusion. Patricia had the same symptoms only more severe. This spreading of our symptoms meant we needed to detoxify both the Watertown apartment and the Red House if we were to have places where we could stay.

Our efforts to neutralize the paint became even more critical. I ordered four more rolls of denny foil, foil tape, and an ozone machine. I used denny foil in Watertown to try to create a safe area in the apartment. Foil on the inside of the bedroom door was to keep out paint fumes while we were sleeping. Foil on the outside of the bedroom door was to prevent paint fumes from entering while we were not in the bedroom. A layer of denny foil between the living room and kitchen was to keep fumes in the kitchen and away from the bedroom. Denny foil over the bathroom door kept fumes in there, but also made entering it more complicated. The door from the kitchen to the back room also had denny foil on both sides. While the denny foil seemed to help, we slept with three air filters on in the bedroom and still had symptoms.

I applied more denny foil in Great Barrington as well. In order to lessen the flow of paint fumes upstairs from the first-floor bathroom, I denny foiled all the walls of the bathroom on the second floor. I also put foil on all walls adjacent to and outside of that bathroom. Trying to make Patricia's bedroom usable again, I put denny foil on its floor and walls.

For a short time thereafter our symptoms seemed to lessen; but when we tried sleeping in Patricia's bedroom once more, we both woke the next morning nearly immobilized by stiff, aching muscles, sore joints, and extreme fatigue. Patricia had to work at the hospital that day. She took seven grams of oral vitamin C and somehow got herself together to go to her job. As the day went on, she felt better outside of the house.

Since denny foiling had not contained the paint toxins, we began intensive ozoning both at the Red House and at the apartment. Although ozoning had failed us twice before, it now seemed our best option. For the next three weeks we spent all our time either working at our jobs or ozoning to make the apartment and the house livable. I was furious that we were paying nearly fifteen hundred dollars rent per month for two residences and yet had no safe place to stay.

Patricia had stopped cooking in Great Barrington, and now we were unable to use the Watertown kitchen, which had been essential for our rotation diet. We were forced to eat in restaurants, which rarely served the organic, pesticide-free food we needed. Restaurants also exposed us to the hazards of other people's perfume, cologne, and hair spray.

To prepare for ozoning in Watertown we cleared the bathroom and kitchen of whatever we did not want exposed to ozone and sealed the cabinets and refrigerator with denny foil and foil tape. It worked best to ozone either the bathroom or the kitchen separately rather than at the same time. We put the ozone machine in the room we were doing, set its timer for two to three hours, sealed the apartment doors, and left. While the machine was on, we went out to eat or sat in the car or went to the office where Patricia worked. We had nowhere else to go.

Several times we fell asleep in the office and woke up after midnight. It was the first time in weeks we had truly rested in a place that was not toxic to us. We returned to the apartment at one o'clock in the morning and aired it out for thirty minutes while we sat outside. By then the ozone level was low enough so we could return safely. We got at most five hours sleep before it was time to wake up for another day of working and ozoning.

When we were not working or ozoning in eastern Massachusetts, we drove to western Massachusetts and did the same there. We made the 260-mile round trip two or three times a week. Patricia changed her schedule at the hospital to one day a week so that we no longer had to stay overnight at the Red House. On days she worked, we woke at two in the morning, prepared for the trip, ate, and drove to Great Barrington. I dropped her off at the hospital by seven and then went to the house. I first aired it out. To ozone the bathroom I closed its window, turned on the ozone machine, and sealed the bathroom door. I ran the machine for three hours,

aired the bathroom out, and then ozoned some more. Periodic airing was said to speed up the process of oxidizing and neutralizing
chemicals.

While ozoning was underway, we had to be out of the house.
Since the most intense ozoning occurred in late February and early
March, the temperature outside was often in the teens or below. On
those days I tried to stay warm either in my car or by going to the
library. The few times I went to the library, a musty smell worsened
my symptoms. When the temperature rose above thirty, I went for
a walk or put a phone outside the house and did dictations.

We also had to do our laundry at the Red House. The smells we
encountered just walking by laundromats made us weak and nauseous. Even if we could have tolerated the inside of a laundromat,
residues from other people's detergents, fabric softeners, and antistatic agents would have contaminated our clothing.

With the effects of the primer, shellac, and paint at the Red
House, the emergence of sensitivities to paint in the apartment, and
the urgency of trying to make these places safe, Patricia and I were
in a state of shock. We now rarely slept more than five hours a
night. When awake, we never rested, never let down our guard. We
were in a constant state of crisis control. We were exhausted and
functioning on autopilot.

Our trips back and forth to western Massachusetts became
increasingly dangerous. We drove through blinding snowstorms in
the mountains, nearly sliding off the road on several occasions.
Patricia and I both dozed off at the wheel more than once.
Fortunately, we never got into an accident. Someone must have
been watching over us.

Not only were we exposed to paint where we lived, but also
at a seemingly endless number of other places. When I went to
the qi gong class again hoping to escape the constant insanity of
our daily lives, I was astounded to find that several rooms in the
building had been freshly painted. My muscle aching, nausea,
confusion, and other symptoms intensified. I could not stay there.
Like Patricia I had to give up going to a class that I had planned

to have help in my healing.

One morning during a utilization review meeting at the guidance center's Watertown office, I suddenly developed nausea, abdominal pain, foot cramping, and a sickening taste in my mouth, symptoms I now associated with paint exposure. When these symptoms persisted, I knew I had to find out what was happening. I discovered the cause of my reaction in the stairway. To my disbelief, a workman with an open can of paint was painting the radiator. I had to leave. I was already sick and to stay any longer would risk becoming much worse. I told my superiors why I had to leave and offered to review charts elsewhere. Failing to understand the seriousness of the situation, they asked me to stay another hour or two; but I refused.

By then the Watertown apartment had improved significantly. Ozoning had been effective and we were able to be there with windows slightly open. When I arrived back at the apartment, I drank several large glasses of water, took six grams of vitamin C, and had a baking soda soak. These measures, together with getting away from the paint, gave me some relief. I later obtained a note from my doctor stating I could not work in that office again until there was a substantial reduction in the level of paint fumes.

Even traveling on the Massachusetts Turnpike exposed me to paint. In the middle of winter, the bathroom stalls in all of the men's rooms at the Turnpike rest areas were being painted. Whenever we made a bathroom stop, I rushed in and out as quickly as possible wearing my charcoal mask to minimize any additional paint exposure.

The previous September I had moved to Great Barrington with a sense of optimism. Now, five months later, my life had become a bizarre battle to survive. Patricia and I had to admit our move to the country was a disaster. We knew we had to do something drastically different if we wanted to get well. We wondered whether anyone had overcome environmental illness. We wanted the torture to stop.

# PART II

# Glimmers of Hope

## March 1991—December 1991

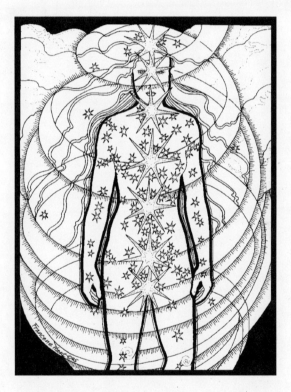

"Something's happening here. What it is
ain't exactly clear."

*Buffalo Springfield*

# CHAPTER FIVE

# Paradoxical Progress

Looking for someone who had overcome environmental illness, I read whatever I could find. Several books by Dr. Sherry Rogers, a specialist in environmental medicine, discussed techniques she had used both in her own recovery from this disorder and in her medical practice. In *Tired or Toxic? A Blueprint for Health,* she explained that following a modified macrobiotic diet helped many people have reduced reactivity to chemicals and less restrictions in their lives. (pp. 314-34) We decided to study more about macrobiotics to see what it might offer us.

The word "macrobiotics" literally means "greater life." Sherry Rogers described it as a "way of eating and living in harmony with nature" with which many people have cured "incurable end-stage cancers." (p.424) The macrobiotic diet was developed and introduced to the United States by the Japanese scholar George Oshwawa in the 1940s and '50s. I first heard of macrobiotics in July of 1970 when I lived in Boston right before starting medical school at the University of Pennsylvania. I attended a lecture given by the now-famous Michio Kushi, George Oshawa's student. I was fascinated by this approach to diet which studied the energies of foods and their effects on health. Following the talk, I bought a macrobiotic cookbook and incorporated some of its recipes into my diet. My exploration of macrobiotics ended that fall amidst the pressures of beginning medical school.

Patricia and I approached this new diet with mixed emotions. On the one hand, it was imperative we find a way to reverse our downward spiral of ever-worsening chemical sensitivities. On the other hand, Patricia had spent months creating a rotation diet she could live with, and had followed it for years. Through extensive research she had collected recipes that she used herself and shared with others in dietary consultations. Although she could not presently cook because of the paint fumes, she had planned to return to her previous cooking style once the kitchens were usable. The macrobiotic diet would be totally different. It would require learning a completely new approach to foods, to cooking, and to meal planning. When she thought about adding this demand to what we already faced, she felt stressed beyond her limits.

To decide what to do, we gathered more information about the benefits of macrobiotics. I read Dr. Anthony Sattilaro's book, *Recalled by Life*, which described his battle with and eventual recovery from prostate cancer. He felt that macrobiotics played a key role in his return to health. Patricia read about macrobiotic cooking. Dr. Sherry Rogers' book, *You Are What You Ate*, described the use of a modified macrobiotic diet to combat chemical sensitivities. The more we read about macrobiotics the more we became convinced it was worth trying. We were having repeated experiences of being passive victims to one chemical exposure after another. Changing our diet was an active step we could take to improve our health.

Although by mid-March we could stay at the Watertown apartment, we kept the windows open as much as possible to maximize ventilation of any chemicals that continued to outgas. As I had done at the Red House, I searched for sources of toxic chemicals and took whatever corrective steps were possible. Since the shellac exposure, we had become sensitive to turpenes, one of its main components. One source of turpenes was pine trees. After discovering unfinished pine in the apartment's kitchen cabinets, I spent hours painstakingly sealing those areas with metal tape and denny foil.

Now that we had a kitchen again, we went ahead with the macrobiotic diet, which was based on eating whole grains, vegetables, beans, and sea vegetables. It focused on the energies of food and how the food was prepared. Since we wanted to heal major illness, we began with the more restrictive macrobiotic healing diet. Sherry Rogers recommended consulting with a macrobiotics counselor who specialized in working with chemically sensitive people. We explored that possibility; but when we were told a consultation would cost hundreds of dollars, we decided to start based on our own research in books.

We began with basic changes, including eliminating dairy products, sugar, sweeteners, desserts, fruit, bread, crackers, and animal protein, except for white fish twice a week. Our dietary staple became whole grains, especially short-grain brown rice. We heightened our awareness of the eating process including chewing each mouthful fifty to one hundred times. The recipes were simple yet time-consuming to prepare and introduced us to many foods we had not eaten before. Of particular importance was the addition of sea vegetables, more commonly called seaweed. Patricia and I were surprised to find that we liked the taste of many of them and were eager to experience their reported effect of removing chemicals from the body.

By early April, we could cope with persistent fumes in the Red House's first-floor bathroom by keeping all the windows wide open while we were there. We then were able to use its large kitchen and sleep there a couple nights a week. The Red House's bigger kitchen gave more room for food preparation. When Patricia was well, cooking had been a passion of hers. She had delighted in preparing and eating international cuisines, particularly Italian, Puerto Rican, and other Latin cultures. By contrast, the macrobiotic healing diet strictly forbade seasonings. Although she found the taste of the food boring, Patricia threw herself into this new cooking style. Now she spent five or more hours a day in the kitchen.

When we began to notice changes in the way we felt, any difficulties starting the macrobiotic diet seemed worthwhile. Within the first several weeks of eating this way, Patricia experienced a clearing of her nearly constant fuzzy-brain feeling. We both noticed increased energy. One morning I awakened to smell the strong odor of pesticides coming from Patricia's breath and skin. Initially, she was repulsed by this phenomenon and embarrassed to be in my presence. She eventually realized the significant potential for getting well this presented.

Not only did strong chemical odors emerge from our skin and mouths, but also in gas expelled from our intestines. We came to call such discharges "detox farts." We first noticed smelly intestinal gas after the paint exposure but did not connect it to the body's attempt to eliminate toxic substances. Later we would have many opportunities to experience our bodies discharging toxins through detox farts. We talked about how belching and farting were considered vulgar in polite western society, but in other cultures they were felt to be part of normal physiology. Now our bodies were making this aspect of their functioning clear to us.

Fortunately, Great Barrington was only a twenty-minute drive from the town of Lee which had a grocery store called "Aveline's," named after Michio Kushi's wife. It specialized in macrobiotic foods and cooking supplies. We spent hundreds of dollars there on food and equipment to start our new diet. Because we were stocking two kitchens, we needed two of everything. We bought two expensive knives imported from Japan for the precise cutting of large quantities of vegetables. Since all the cut vegetables had to be kept separate prior to cooking, we bought twenty small dishes.

We also needed new kinds of equipment, including pickle presses and hand grinders. Macrobiotics stressed that how food was handled during preparation influenced its effect when eaten. According to macrobiotics, electricity had a disruptive effect on the energy of food and any food grinding had to be done by hand. From that perspective, cooking with an electric stove was deviating from macrobiotic teaching, but we knew we could not tolerate a gas stove. In any case, we did not have one. Since Patricia prepared five or more dishes for many meals, the four burners on the stove were no longer enough. We bought five portable electric burners and used them as needed.

Within a month, Patricia felt more comfortable with the basics of macrobiotic cooking. All whole grains and beans were washed meticulously. Vegetables were cut in a precise manner according to the recipe. Patricia could now prepare a number of individual dishes well, but found it challenging and frustrating to combine them into a meal that tasted good to her. The recipes in her macrobiotic cookbooks did not focus on the healing diet; they used fermented products for flavoring. As a compromise, Patricia served mildly seasoned miso soup.

When Patricia needed a break from cooking, we went to a macrobiotic restaurant. Dining out was always problematic. We were continually amazed by how strong other people's perfume, cologne, hair spray, or laundry detergent smelled to us and wondered how they stood the odors themselves. At the restaurant we sat in the no-smoking section as far away from others as possible. If we became aware of odors wafting toward us, we repositioned our chairs or moved to another table to avoid them. Someone unaware of what we were doing might have thought we were engaged in a strange dance.

Eating at the restaurant gave us the opportunity to sample a variety of macrobiotic dishes. When she found the restaurant's miso soup was stronger than hers, Patricia increased the amount of miso she used at home. She came to love her miso soup and ate several bowls at a meal. When I commented on how much miso soup she ate, Patricia replied that she could not stand the lack of flavor and that she needed to enjoy her meals.

During our second month on the diet we told the manager of Aveline's about our progress. Although we continued to have greater mental clarity and to release toxins, muscle aching and fatigue persisted and our chemical sensitivities grew worse. He suggested we were eating too many "contracting" foods and recommended we decrease our intake of miso. He also commented proudly that macrobiotic people were among the most sensitive people in the world. Patricia and I looked at each other with alarm. If that were the case, what were we doing on this diet? We wanted to lessen our sensitivities so that we could have a normal life. Not knowing what else to do, we continued on the diet anyway. Patricia was erratic about her use of miso and closed her ears to my suggestion that she was addicted to it.

With warmer weather we faced new problems. According to our lease we were responsible for maintaining the grounds of the Red House. The landlord had provided a gasoline-powered lawnmower, but we had him remove it from the basement the previous fall. At first I thought I would enjoy mowing the grass. It would be a chance to be outdoors and drink in the beauty of the surrounding mountains. In order to do it myself without exposure to gasoline fumes, I bought an electric-powered mower and a long extension cord. With these purchases I began to have feelings of accomplishment. After numerous failures, here was one problem it appeared I had been able to solve.

This sense of accomplishment was short-lived. Soon after I started mowing, I began feeling confused and disoriented. My muscles ached and I had a taste in my mouth. Disregarding these symptoms, I continued for twenty minutes. I then went into the house for water and told Patricia what had happened. She recalled her doctor telling her that cut grass contains turpenes, the same substance found in shellac. In the process of cutting the grass I was surrounding myself with one of the substances which poisoned us three months earlier. In the past I had enjoyed the smell of cut grass, now it was another hazard to my health.

Patricia wanted me to stop mowing right away. At first I was too invested in succeeding to listen to her. Over the next three weekends I tried various approaches to cutting the grass. I wore my charcoal mask and cotton gloves. To minimize the amount of exposure at any one time I alternated ten minutes mowing with ten minutes resting. Even with these approaches I was not symptom-free. I needed longer and longer intervals before I felt able to resume. The grass grew faster than I could keep up with. Finally, I had to admit defeat again. As routine an activity as mowing the lawn became one more area of my life that was out of my control.

Now I needed to hire someone to do the yard work but had no

idea where to find them. We had been so busy with daily survival issues that we had met few local residents. When I hired Harold to work for us one Saturday, he was accompanied by his brother-in-law, Chris, a recent addition to the growing ranks of laid-off workers in western Massachusetts. Upon seeing the overgrown yard, Chris expressed interest in mowing the lawn. We discussed a price and agreed he would do it every week or two as needed. I stipulated that in order for him to use his gasoline-powered mower, he would mow on days when we were not there. As repeatedly happened with environmental illness, I had tried to solve one chemical problem (the gasoline-powered lawnmower) by buying something else (the electric lawnmower), and my attempted solution had failed. I was left with both the electric lawnmower, which I could not use, and the expense of paying to have the lawn mowed.

Although we followed the macrobiotic diet, took supplements, and had acupuncture and massage, our sensitivities continued to worsen. By early June, we no longer could tolerate sleeping in Patricia's bedroom even with the windows open. Previously, it had been the best room in the house for us. We did not know why it was no longer all right and were unsure what to do. I remembered an old canvas tent that three medical school classmates and I used during a trip to the Rockies in 1973. Perhaps Patricia and I could sleep outdoors in it. We both had enjoyed camping but never dreamed we would need to resort to sleeping in a tent because we could not tolerate the inside of our house.

During our next trip to Watertown, I retrieved the all-canvas, two-person tent from the deep recesses of my bedroom closet. After being aired out, it smelled surprisingly good, even though it had not been used in six years. I found an ideal location for the tent on a gentle slope in front of the house facing the mountains. That night I brought out bedding, and we slept under the stars. It had been too long since I had slept so close to the earth and sky. Both of us felt better sleeping outside than sleeping in the house. We awakened the next morning feeling more refreshed than we had in months.

Throughout the summer, we slept in the tent as much as possi-

ble, but having the outdoors for our bedroom brought its own problems. We discovered that even when Chris mowed the day before
we arrived, turpenes in the cuttings made us sick. I requested he cut
the grass two days before we returned to the Red House. We did
much better on that schedule.

Our closest neighbors were a retired investment banker and
his wife, who lived an eighth of a mile away. We became so sen-
sitized to grass cuttings that their cuttings also started to affect us.
Putting myself in as positive a frame of mind as possible, I called
the banker and told him about the symptoms we had after his lawn
was mowed. I said it would help us if his lawn was done earlier in
the week, but I would understand if he could not make that
change. Although he seemed irritated by my request, he agreed to
see what his landscaper could do. When their lawn was cut earlier in the week, Patricia and I had fewer symptoms in the tent.
When their lawn was cut the day we arrived, we had worse muscle aching and fatigue.

The banker said nothing to me, but I later learned from Jacob
our neighbor's true thoughts. He complained to Jacob that we
seemed rather fussy. I told Jacob it was not a matter of being fussy,
it was a matter of trying to survive when a growing number of substances made us sick at ever greater distances.

Even with our continually increasing sensitivities we tried to
take advantage of the magnificent natural surroundings as much as
possible. We discovered the hidden treasure of Mt. Everett State
Park, a twenty-minute drive from our house. The park had dense
woods and a dirt road going three-quarters of the way up the mountain. Halfway up was a peaceful lake that had its own resident
beaver. Hawks flew overhead. On top of the mountain were beautiful views south to the Litchfield Hills of Connecticut and west to
the Catskill Mountains of New York. At first the dirt road was
closed to vehicular traffic. We rarely saw other people and imagined it to be our own mountain.

Patricia and I both felt better on the mountain top, particularly
with a strong breeze blowing to help clear our bodies of the chem-

icals that continued to plague us. Patricia's generalized joint and muscle pain and weakness were so great that often she had to drag herself up the mountain or forgo the trip altogether. My muscles were sore and tight, but I still managed to hike to the top three times a week. We felt so much better up there that we fantasized about how we could live in such a location.

The healing quality of Mt. Everett changed in early June. Heavy equipment brought in dirt and regraded the road, which was opened to traffic two-thirds of the way up the mountain. Climbing it now often involved confronting motor vehicles and their exhaust fumes. When we managed to avoid the exhaust, we were surprised by yet another source of toxins near the top.

Caught in a summer downpour, we were relieved to reach a wooden shelter and be able to dry out. While sitting there, I became nauseous and developed muscle spasms. Something was wrong. When I looked around, I noticed fresh paint. Even on a mountain in a state park we had again encountered paint. Filled with anger, I questioned why people could not leave well enough alone. What was someone else's idea of improvement was for us another toxic exposure. Having recognized the problem, we left and walked out into the pouring rain. Thereafter, we kept our distance from the shelter.

There was nowhere Patricia and I could find a safe haven. Our efforts to improve our health by changing our diet had yet to succeed. We were running out of ideas as to what to try next.

# CHAPTER SIX

# Deepening Desperation

June marked nine months of unceasing effort to make the Red House livable. Instead of feeling better, we grew progressively worse. In addition to generalized myalgia and aching joints which made moving painful, Patricia began having more frequent episodes of extreme weakness. At those times, it took all of her energy to continue standing and finish what she was doing. When she could stand no longer, Patricia often crawled up the stairs, fell on her bed, and cried herself to sleep. She complained of persistent headaches, nausea, and dizziness. We both were troubled by cloudy thinking and confusion. The muscles of my arms, legs, and back felt so tight they seemed ready to snap.

In light of our steady deterioration, we asked why we kept returning to Great Barrington. The answer was we had nowhere else to go. The Red House was the only place we had found where it seemed possible to get better. We had already spent thousands of dollars trying to make it habitable for us. I worried about not being able to afford another move and the cost of making another place "safe." If we failed where we were, where would we go?

Throughout the summer, I tried harder to make the Red House free of toxins. We were certain something there was poisoning us. I hoped that once the cause was identified and eliminated, our healing would begin.

Our symptoms guided my search for hazards. Since Patricia's bouts of extreme fatigue, which we called "collapsing," occurred mainly in the kitchen, I started there. Close examination revealed a strong draft from the adjoining family room, which was filled with unpacked boxes. We thought chemicals from the boxes might account for Patricia's prostration. She remembered similar past episodes that followed formaldehyde exposure. After I spent two days furiously taking all the boxes out of the family room and dumping their contents in what were to have been Patricia's exercise room and my office, she felt better; but within a week the spells returned full force.

These episodes in the kitchen occurred most often near the sink. Since we had already detoxified that area, I turned my attention to the basement below. I found plywood and other building supplies that contained large amounts of formaldehyde and other chemicals. I immediately began taking them to a shed on the far side of the property. Over that weekend, I removed five wheelbarrows and three station wagons full of toxic items. Eliminating them improved the air quality in the basement but made no difference in the kitchen.

When I worked in the basement for a long time, I too felt weak and exhausted. I could hardly walk, as if I were moving through sludge. I felt like collapsing. The only way I could continue was to alternate fifteen minutes working with fifteen minutes resting outdoors.

Since my symptoms in the basement matched Patricia's in the kitchen, I looked there carefully for problems. With the construction materials out of the way, more of the basement was visible. During the next heavy storm I checked to see whether any rain came in and was infuriated to find water entering in four places. At two sites it gushed out of the wall as if pouring out of a leaking dam.

After the storm, most of the cellar was dry, but the southeast corner remained wet. I noticed the adjacent wooden storage platform's supports had watermarks and were rotten. When I lifted one of its planks, I was horrified to find a stagnant pool of water. The underside of the board was covered with mold. Panicked and enraged by what I saw, I ripped out the remaining planks, rushed them outside, and threw them down.

The clatter of the boards startled Patricia who raced out to see what the noise was. I told her what I had found, and we both stood there in disbelief. We had been anxious about mold when we first looked at the house and saw its wet basement. Based on the landlord's assurance the basement was dry and comments by the realtor and others that any wetness could be managed, we had signed the lease. Now we brooded over the harmful effects of this chronic mold exposure.

I called Jacob who expressed surprise about the rotting storage platform. He said initially it held valuable works of art. I told him anything stored there now would be ruined. Although I had fretted over his response to my tearing out the storage shelf, he accepted my actions as an attempt to make the house safe.

Jacob and I also discussed other improvements for the basement. When I told him about the water, he agreed to have Harold fix any problems that were simple and inexpensive to repair. I suggested the house's lack of gutters was one cause of leakage in the basement. He replied there had been gutters years ago, but he tore them down after they became clogged with pine needles. Jacob agreed to install low-cost gutters on certain sections of the roof to reduce water pressure on the foundation.

While waiting for Harold to make repairs, I did what I could. I removed an old bookcase from beside the north wall and behind it found piles of moldy-smelling black dirt. I carted out two wheelbarrows full. When Patricia looked in a nearby child's play stove, she was shocked to find large mushrooms growing. Not only was the basement wet, but it was also a veritable haven for fungi! I got rid of the stove and the mushrooms.

Some parts of the basement were more difficult to fix. With the bookcase out of the way, I saw a three-foot-long, horizontal crack in the north wall. When I reported it to Jacob, he informed me of his plan to redo that part of the foundation during extensive renovations in the future. This piece of information awakened us to the realization that the house had significant structural defects which would be a continuing source of major mold contamination in the basement and throughout the house. However, if these renovations were done, we would not be able to tolerate the chemicals involved.

Here was another dilemma of environmental illness to which we had become accustomed. We repeatedly identified problems and tried to solve them, but the solutions only caused more difficulties. Eliminating the problems in the basement would entail exposure to harmful substances and would likely worsen our health. With our bodies' functioning so badly impaired, we no longer had healthy options but merely choices among least-toxic alternatives. For the present, Jacob could not afford renovations. I cleaned the basement and tried to keep it dry.

Although the Red House was supposed to be a place of rest and recovery, we never had time to rest. Patricia continued to spend most of her time buying food, preparing it, and doing dishes. I worked nonstop to make the house safe. Periodically I ozoned the first-floor bathroom, but it still made us sick. As a result, we sealed it off from the rest of the house. I repeatedly ozoned my yet-to-be-slept-in bedroom but to no avail. I even had special low-toxicity paint applied in an attempt to seal in fumes from paint put on the previous December. Unfortunately, that room still evoked symptoms, and we had to keep it closed off as well.

My search for why we felt sick in Patricia's bedroom led to the suspicious attic storage space entered through a doorway in the east wall. Although Jacob had asked us to keep out of the attic, we were now locked in a life-and-death battle with the house. I needed to know if anything in there was aggravating our condition. After I pried the door open, a strong, bitter odor assaulted me, causing muscle aching, fatigue, and confusion. I was reacting to something but did not know what.

We had a huge problem. The attic's many contents appeared to be hazardous to us; but since they belonged to the landlord, I could not get rid of them. As an alternative, I decided to seal the attic off from the rest of the house.

Over the next two weekends, I emptied out the attic, lined it with denny foil, and then put everything back. I found numerous harmful items, including cleaning fluid, furniture polish, moldy-smelling clothes, clothes smelling of dry cleaning chemicals, foam mattresses, and other things. With so many toxins right next door, I understood why Patricia and I never could relax and feel symptom-free in her bedroom.

This attic project epitomized life with environmental illness, that is, constantly being poisoned and attacked. Although I tried to physically pace myself, I became exhausted and was slowed by diffuse muscle aching. I came across skeletons of dead mice and wasps nesting in the gables. As I carried out a framed print, I was stung by a wasp. I stumbled over a rolled-up rug and hit the floor. The glass in the frame broke, slicing my arm. As I rushed to clean my wound, I screamed that nothing I did worked out anymore and wondered how I had fallen to such a wretched state. When I finally sealed the attic door, I was relieved the project was done.

I also tried to create a safe, dry place for us to sleep. We spent most nights outdoors in the tent but needed a dry option for when it rained. I first draped a tarpaulin made of plastic drop cloths over the tent. This system performed adequately in a light mist but failed miserably in a downpour.

Next I turned to the family room, which had been cleared of boxes earlier in the summer. Although the room was empty, we had not used it because of a strong, acrid odor that made my joints ache. For days I cleaned it trying to eliminate that smell. I hoped using the tent on dry nights and the family room on wet ones would let us sleep comfortably in any weather.

A heavy rain soon put this plan to the test. We placed a new organic cotton futon I had bought on the concrete floor in the family room and left two windows open for ventilation. Tired from endless physical activity, I easily fell asleep. When I woke up at five the next morning, all my joints ached. My hands were particularly stiff and painful. The family room was not safe for me. It was another room to avoid.

The trap of environmental illness continued to tighten its grip. It even interfered with acupuncture treatments. We had been going to Kiiko at the acupuncture school in Watertown. Each appointment brought the challenge of finding an office I could tolerate. One evening as I lay down on the treatment table to relax, my muscles suddenly tightened all over. I felt light-headed and had a disgusting taste in my mouth. Something was very wrong.

In a panic I looked around the office and noticed a new container. When I picked it up, I smelled bleach. Bleach, which made me weak and nauseous, was now in every treatment room at the acupuncture school. New state regulations required that it be used daily to wipe down equipment. Staying there would be too dangerous; I had to leave. I felt disheartened and disgusted that my illness had blocked another avenue to healing.

August was a most difficult month. Patricia and I were sicker than the year before, when we moved to the country to escape environmental illness. We had many more sensitivities and kept six of the house's eight rooms sealed to avoid toxic exposures. Even the natural surroundings caused problems.

Every afternoon at four, like clockwork, our symptoms became more pronounced, including increased muscle aching, confusion, and fatigue. Our reading led us to conclude that mold spores released at that time likely caused this daily aggravation. We coped by trying to be indoors with the windows closed between four and seven in the afternoon and by running four air filters full blast.

At the same time our lives were becoming more and more constricted, we had to decide what to do. Should we renew the house lease which ended in September? Should we move? Patricia begged me to leave everything behind and move into a porcelain trailer, a hypoallergenic dwelling to which people with environmental illness retreat as a last resort. I refused. I emphasized the difficulty we had finding a place which met our criteria, the expense of moving, and the money already spent to make this house safe. I expressed hope that improvement was just ahead. While I argued for staying, I had little confidence in that option. In fact, I was anxious about remaining and terrified by what moving would entail.

Changes in Watertown further intensified the pressures on us,

making it impossible even to think about moving. Although the population in my six-unit apartment building had been stable for years, three units adjacent to mine were vacated at the same time. My landlord, Glen, now wanted to renovate them, a prospect we dreaded. We had come to rely on the apartment as our place of relatively less chemical exposure indoors. Glen's plans threatened this limited safety.

As I searched frantically for a way out of our latest predicament, I encountered other chemically sensitive individuals who had faced similar situations. One of them, Rose, described how she had taken her landlord to court in order to stop him from painting the apartment building where she lived. She told me about my rights as a person disabled by chemical sensitivities. While she willingly provided this information, she indicated she was too preoccupied with her own problems to offer any other assistance.

Heartened by my talk with Rose, I spoke with Glen. I told him about my illness and the need to have less toxic products used in any work he did. He hesitated at first but then agreed, especially when I offered to pay any extra cost. Since he wanted to paint right away, I had the special products sent from Texas by next day air at a cost of an additional hundred dollars. Although low-toxicity paint and joint compound were used, Patricia and I reacted to them for weeks until they dried and gassed out.

While our health continued to deteriorate, we worried about our jobs. Expenses remained high as we followed the lifestyle we had been told would help us get better, but chemical sensitivities and fatigue increasingly interfered with our ability to work. If a patient wore strong-smelling perfume, my muscles tightened all over, and I struggled to think clearly. Cologne, perfume, and hair spray worn by other staff members caused symptoms and made attending meetings distressing. Patricia tolerated the environment of the coronary care unit in Great Barrington; but when the census there was low, she was asked to work elsewhere in the hospital. She had to decline because those areas had been remodeled. Whenever that issue came up, her job stability seemed tenuous.

I had to fight to be able to keep working at the guidance center. Overall the environment there had been manageable, but in August the administration proposed changes which endangered my health. They wanted me to move my office from one side of the building to the other. After a brief inspection of the new office revealed several hazards, I protested. The office I had used for twelve years was tolerable, and I wanted to keep it. When pressured from above to switch, I sought legal advice.

I learned that because of my disability, my employer was obliged to make reasonable accommodations for me and that it would be to my advantage to show willingness to resolve the conflict. With that in mind, I removed plastic objects and other harmful items from the proposed office. Then I smelled mold. I found mold stains on the rug and a crack in the foundation where water had leaked in. Based on these findings, I refused that room. I told my boss I would switch, but any new office would have to be safe for me. I then worried about my superiors' response to the stance I had taken. Once again I was forced to tell people in positions of authority what I needed, despite my fears about their reactions. Much later I would appreciate these experiences as an important teaching which my illness offered me.

As the stress level continued to escalate, it reached unbearable proportions. There were major problems in both living situations and at work. We had to decide about the lease. In hope of gaining relief, we again went to Kiiko for acupuncture, this time to her house in Natick. With our demanding schedules it was hard to find appointment times. We finally arranged to see her Monday mornings on the trip from Great Barrington to Boston.

When we went to Kiiko's house the next week, I was surprised to meet Eli Jacobe, who was leaving as we arrived. Eli practiced acupuncture in Rockport and assisted Kiiko at the acupuncture school. In the past he and I had exchanged ideas and resources about energetic approaches to healing. Because of my sickness, we had not spoken in over a year. After I described my plight, Eli told me about a physicist named Steven Rochlitz who claimed to have

cured himself of environmental illness using energy-balancing techniques. He had written a book entitled *Allergies and Candida with the Physicist's Rapid Solution*. Eli offered to send me a copy to look at. I thanked him for his help and we said good-bye.

Walking into Kiiko's office, I pondered the synchronicity of this meeting. Just as Patricia and I had run out of things to try, I met Eli. We had not seen each other in months, and now he had told me about someone who had cured himself of environmental illness. Patricia and I were sicker than ever and stuck in our efforts to get well, but I had not given up. I eagerly awaited Rochlitz's book and the possibility of a way for Patricia and me to regain our health.

Anticipation of learning how someone had overcome environmental illness made the week pass quickly. When we arrived in Great Barrington on Thursday, the package from Eli was waiting. I ripped it open and began reading. My attention was drawn to chapter one, "A Physicist at Death's Door." As I read Rochlitz's story of suffering for years with symptoms which were finally diagnosed as environmental illness, I knew his life had been a living hell as ours had become. Frustrated by standard medical treatments, Rochlitz explored alternative healing modalities and eventually studied kinesiology. Within that framework he devised the energy-balancing techniques which eliminated his life-long allergies. Thereafter, chemicals no longer bothered him.

Inspired by Rochlitz's book, I wanted to know more about what he had done. The address on the copyright page indicated he was located in Mahopac, New York, a two-hour drive from Great Barrington. When I called, Steven answered. He spoke slowly in a heavy New York accent. After telling him briefly about Patricia and myself, I asked if he could help us. He replied without question that he could. I wanted to see him right away, but the earliest available appointments were a week later. In the meantime, he recommended we do the exercises in his book to balance our bodies' energies and improve our functioning.

The next week was busier than usual. My friend, Les Gundry, visited from Philadelphia for the weekend. We had met during my internship at Bryn Mawr Hospital where he was the medical librarian. We shared common interests in travel and spiritual studies but had not seen each other in years. Given Philadelphia's closer proximity to Great Barrington than to Boston, he decided to make the trip.

I prepared Les for the visit by telling him about chemicals that Patricia and I needed to avoid because of our sensitivities. He was taken aback by my discussion of the toxicity of shampoo, hair conditioner, cologne, and deodorant but agreed to avoid using scented products. Les went by train to New York City and then to Hudson, New York, where I met him and drove him back to Great Barrington. We were glad to see each other, but he expressed concern about my gaunt appearance. With a height of five feet, eight inches, I now weighed one hundred fifteen pounds, down from my previous weight of one hundred thirty. During the hour drive to Great Barrington, we talked about our recent experiences. Les told me about his trip to Eastern Europe and the Soviet Union. I told him about my daily struggle to survive.

When we arrived at the Red House, I introduced Les to Patricia, who was busy cooking a macrobiotic dinner. I had told him about our new diet, which he was willing to try except for the seaweed. Les marveled at the house and its surroundings. Since Patricia and I slept in the tent, he would sleep in her bedroom. He rested there briefly after his trip. When I went to tell him dinner was ready, both Patricia and I were anxious to learn how he felt in the bedroom. He said the room was refreshing and the mountain air invigorating.

Les' ease in the room that made us ill confused and frightened Patricia. She had a fleeting awareness that the problem was not in the room but inside us. She remembered moments of collapsing when it had occurred to her that if she were endangered by fire she would be able to move. At those times she pondered the true source of her immobility. Later she told me such thoughts led her to question her sanity. At the time she said nothing.

Over the next two days, I took Les to art museums and historical sites which he wanted to visit. Previously, I had enjoyed that kind of activity, but now I was uncertain about my ability to make it through the outings. Patricia did not even try.

Les and I went to a Winslow Homer exhibit at the Sterling and Francine Clark Art Institute in Williamstown. The exhibit received rave reviews, and I wanted to see it even before I knew he was coming. When we entered the museum, though, I discovered all the galleries had new carpet. Soon I developed muscle aching and dizziness. I told Les I could not stay very long. After racing through the exhibit in less than ten minutes, I sat outdoors for two hours waiting for him. I wanted to spend more time viewing the paintings, but the carpet's chemicals were too much for me. Here was one more example of how my illness cut me off from life.

The next day we went to the Norman Rockwell Museum in Stockbridge. I had driven by it many times on trips between Great Barrington and Boston. Although I wanted to see it, I was always too busy. Les' visit seemed the perfect time to go. As we approached the ticket window, there were crowds of people inside and outside the museum. After Les bought his ticket, I told the cashier about my chemical sensitivities and asked if I could first check how I felt inside. She agreed. As soon as I entered the crowded foyer, I was assaulted by the smells of hair sprays, perfumes, and colognes. Instantly, I developed muscle cramping, confusion, and a chemical taste in my mouth. Barely mustering enough strength to wave to get Les' attention, I then stumbled out the front door. I told him staying any longer would be perilous for me. I suggested he tour the museum and then call me at the Red House when he was done.

As I drove home alone, I felt crushed by the events of the last two days. Les' visit had encouraged me to again try activities which I previously enjoyed. My failed attempts underscored how much my health had deteriorated. I wanted to go to museums and to pursue other interests, but my reactions made it impossible for me to do so. I no longer could live life as most people think of it. I felt like a canary from the coal mines of old, merely an indicator of the toxic effects of chemicals all around me.

Three hours later Les called, and I went to pick him up. He thoroughly enjoyed the museum. He said the ticket seller told him I should come back some day when the museum first opened if I wanted to avoid the crowds. I never did visit the Rockwell Museum during our nineteen months in the Berkshires.

Later that afternoon Patricia and I drove Les to the train station in Hudson. As we said good-bye, he told me how worried he was about me. Never before had he seen me in such a debilitated state. He added that he would pray for me. I felt I would need divine intervention to emerge from this frightening and perplexing tangle of reactions and symptoms.

On Monday we renewed the lease for the Red House, mainly because we were too tired and too busy to do otherwise. We had no idea how we would make it through another year there, but we had nowhere else to go. Patricia agreed to the renewal partly because she remembered her psychotherapist telling her she tended to try to resolve difficulties by running away from them. In fact, Patricia had moved twelve times in the last thirteen years. She was ready to try something different. I also knew we needed to try something other than what we had been doing for the last fifteen months if we wanted to regain our health and our lives. We hoped the consultations with Steven Rochlitz on Friday would open the way to healing.

# CHAPTER SEVEN

# New Frameworks
# for Healing

We awakened early Friday morning as the sun's first rays peeked over the mountains, filling our tent with light. A year earlier to the day we had driven to Great Barrington to finalize arrangements for renting the Red House. Now we had to keep most of it closed off. The reason for our continued symptoms was not clear but seemed related to toxins in and around the house as well as to our impaired immune systems. Today we would travel again, this time to appointments with Steven Rochlitz, the physicist who claimed to have cured himself of symptoms even worse than ours. We looked to him for a new approach to stop our downward spiral of ever-worsening sensitivities. We desperately wanted to regain our health.

It was a struggle to get going in the morning. In the past, I had awakened early and then meditated or done whatever else I wanted to do, but for months I had been slowed down. Patricia had experienced difficulty waking up for years, and now the problem was worse. Having environmental illness meant that everything we did took longer. There was the usual routine of cooking a whole-grain breakfast from scratch and then preparing lunch to go. No restaurant on the way to Mahopac would have the organic, whole-grain meals of a macrobiotic diet. While Patricia cooked a dish of squash, millet, onions, and cauliflower and loaded it into thermos bottles, I collected other items for the trip, including several quarts of filtered water. An hour later than planned, the station wagon was packed, and I sped down our half-mile-long driveway en route to New York.

We spent the first half of the trip yelling at each other. I complained we were always late and I ended up having to hurry wherever we went. No matter how much planning we did, there was always another reaction or another set of symptoms which came up that had to be dealt with before we could leave. Patricia griped that all she did was cook and all her cooking was not helping us get better. We both felt constantly frustrated by the limitations we repeatedly encountered.

The last half of the trip was spent in silent anger and anticipation. We wondered what our sessions would be like. Would we have as good a response as Steven said he had? Was it really possible to overcome environmental illness? My life for fifteen months had focused on trying to keep myself safe by avoiding toxic substances, a task I had learned was impossible. In fact, it seemed the more I tried avoiding chemicals, the more I became entangled in other reactions and developed more symptoms. Patricia had lived this pattern for years but said it had been manageable before she met me.

We left so late that I worried about arriving for our appointments on time; but driving fast without any stops, we were there a few minutes early. After hastily eating lunch in the car, we went to the door and met Steven, a large, tall man with an imposing presence. He invited us into his living room where he began the consultation.

Steven took a detailed history first from me, then from Patricia. He repeatedly asked why I was so thin. When he heard we were following a macrobiotic diet, he strongly suggested stopping it. He said, in his experience, people who were universal reactors had an underlying Candida problem that would be exacerbated by eating fermented foods and a diet rich in grains. Medical researchers beginning with Orin Truss have argued for the role played by the yeast, *Candida albicans*, in chronic illness. While Candida occurs normally in human intestines, Truss and others have found that Candida overgrowth can produce far-ranging effects throughout the body resulting in numerous health problems.

We had considered the possibility of our having a Candida imbalance but had come up with no firm evidence in that regard. Previous blood tests Patricia had for Candida were negative. In light of her health problems, her doctor suggested an anti-Candida diet anyway. As a result, the rotation diet Patricia had followed for years included avoiding sweets and fermented foods and limiting carbohydrates. Although we both felt better initially when we started the rotation diet, the improvement did not last; and we each eventually turned our focus to eliminating chemicals from our environment. Patricia began suspecting Candida was again a problem when she noticed a thick coating on her tongue shortly before the consultation with Steven. His comments heightened her concerns.

After an hour of history taking, Steven led us to his treatment room. While Patricia watched, he began assessing me. His primary means of investigation was kinesiology, a biofeedback technique that uses changes in muscle strength to access information about the body.

Through a system that he developed, Steven evaluated me for sensitivity to several chemicals and for the adverse effects of a variety of organisms. His findings indicated I was sensitive to formaldehyde and acetaldehyde and had problems with excess Candida and with the energetically disruptive effects of Candida, which he termed "Candida energy imbalance." He reminded me his testing worked at the level of the body's energies and suggested I might want to obtain laboratory tests from my physician to confirm his findings.

Steven then assessed the functioning and integration of my nervous system and energy body. In nearly every case I initially tested weak. He said such results were common in people with Candida and/or environmental illness. For each item on which I was weak, he had me do a correction that involved resting my hands on various acupuncture points or moving in a particular way. Then he retested. The process was remarkable. Each correction resulted in improvement. By the time we were done, I felt completely differ-

ent. I had a greater sense of balance, a clearer head, and more energy than I had felt for months. What a relief to feel better! I was
speechless.

Next it was Patricia's turn. Steven went through the same pro-
cedures he had done with me. She tested weak on several ecological factors, including Candida. Steven then tested for imbalances in
functioning and showed her corrections as indicated. Throughout
the session Patricia also noticed definite changes in how she felt.
Her head became much clearer. In fact, for the first time in years
she felt clearheaded. She also was aware of her legs and feet and
suddenly recognized that for years she had not really felt them. Her
back, which had been tight and sore, was more relaxed. She noticed
changes in her spatial orientation. After some corrections she felt
taller, after others shorter or wider. Overall she was more in her
body. By the end of the session Patricia felt like a different person.
She, too, was surprised by the improvement that had occurred.

Before we left, Steven recommended we consider the role that
mold sensitivities might be playing in our deteriorating health. He
again urged us to stop the macrobiotic diet and to resume the yeast-
free diet. He advised doing the exercises in his book regularly. He
also mentioned he was teaching an eleven-day seminar in
November, which would include much of what he used in his work.
Based on our response to the consultations, I expressed interest. I
was unsure how I would manage the logistics of attending the training but wanted to explore doing it. In the meantime, Patricia and I
could see how we responded to his approach over time.

During the two-hour trip back to Great Barrington, we discussed our sessions and talked about changes we wanted to make.
We decided to modify our diet by eliminating fermented foods,
rotating grains, and gradually adding animal protein, which we also
rotated. We wanted to seek out and eliminate any mold in our
house.

When I surveyed the house, I was surprised by how much mold
was present even with the cleaning we had done already. The
drainage tray under the refrigerator was covered with a thick layer

of black, smelly mold which I removed using gloves and a charcoal mask. We felt better after it was gone.

Next we noticed a mold smell coming from the radiator in the kitchen. I cleaned the radiator as well as I could, but the smell persisted. Closer inspection revealed the smell came from floor boards under the radiator. I pondered how to eliminate that mold. Bleach would kill it but would also make us very sick. When I learned about a machine that controlled mold by emitting grapefruit seed extract, I bought four of them for a thousand dollars and placed one next to the radiator and the others around the house. Still, the smell under the kitchen radiator did not completely go away.

Another area of concern was Patricia's bedroom. It connected to the attic storage space which I had worked on four months earlier. With winter coming, soon we would not be able to sleep in the tent. Her bedroom offered the best prospect for a relatively safe place to sleep, but we needed first to get rid of any mold there. Toward this end, we decided to ozone again.

Although we had limited success neutralizing chemicals with the ozone machine, ozone was said to be effective at killing mold. To prepare for this process we moved furniture from Patricia's room into my yet-to-be-used bedroom. I moved my clothing from her closet onto a table in the living room. Wanting to avoid adding clutter to the mess we had already, Patricia chose to put her clothes in my bedroom wrapped in a barrier cloth and denny foil. We then ozoned for four-hour intervals and aired the room out in between.

The next afternoon we moved the furniture back into Patricia's bedroom. When she looked for a clean shirt, she put on one that had been in my room. Patricia was panicked by instant muscle spasms in her neck and shoulders. Her clothing had been in my bedroom, wrapped in the protective barrier, for only a day. The room had been painted three months earlier with "safe" paint and ten months earlier with regular paint and baking soda. She was stunned to find that now all her clothing was contaminated by paint fumes and she could not tolerate any of it. The only clothing unaffected was what she had on and a few items in the laundry basket. Her need to minimize the chaos while we tried to make her bedroom safe had left her with an entire wardrobe she could not wear.

Patricia's emotions ranged from panic to disbelief. She questioned how this could have happened. How was she so sensitive that clothes left for twenty-four hours wrapped in a vapor barrier in a room painted months earlier had become unwearable? She found it difficult to believe she had nothing to wear. She felt like she was going crazy. We already had enough trouble trying to survive. Depressed and scared, I worried about how we would cope with this latest disaster of Patricia, in effect, losing her entire wardrobe.

We both wondered why whatever we did to make the house better ended up creating a worse mess. The whole scenario was so bizarre, so unbelievable. Patricia screamed and yelled that in the five years with environmental illness before meeting me, she had never seen anything like the sequence of disasters we had gone through since we decided to live together to get better. She then started to calm down as she heard a quiet voice inside her saying everything would be all right and there was a reason for all this. Alternating between hysteria and tranquillity, she began to look at what to do next.

We added efforts to retrieve Patricia's paint-tainted clothing to our already full schedules. She washed everything several times, dried it, and then hung it outside to air. When she tried the clothing on again, she developed extreme muscle spasms, especially in her upper back and shoulders. Although she could not smell paint any more, clearly there still were chemicals in the clothing which produced these symptoms. She washed it in Super Clean hoping that would remove the chemicals, but the clothing remained unwearable. She became increasingly fearful that she would have nothing of her own to wear. She knew she could not tolerate going into a clothing store or wearing new clothes.

Patricia felt completely stripped of her identity as an attractive woman. She recalled how she used to be so particular about her appearance. She had regularly gotten her hair permed and enjoyed fussing with her makeup. She had loved putting on Chanel No. 5

perfume and dressing up to go out to dinner, but her sensitivities changed all that. Her last perm in 1989 coincided with such severe muscle spasms in her back that she was out of work for two months. Using perfume was out of the question. She stopped wearing make-up soon after we moved to Great Barrington when I complained about the smell of her mascara. Now her clothing was ruined and the only things she could wear were my shirt and jeans and one jumper we had managed to salvage.

I had clothing problems of my own. For over a year, I had been unable to wear new clothes because of reactions to chemicals in them. The clothes I could tolerate were wearing away. I was going into the second winter of being unable to wear sport coats to the office. The sweater I wore in place of them now had holes in both elbows.

We continued practicing the exercises Steven showed us. They helped, but their effects wore off; and we had to repeat them several times a day. Although Patricia saw that the corrections worked, she needed frequent reminders to do them. Having lived a long time in a resigned state of hopelessness about her illness, she had trouble viewing herself as having the knowledge and ability to change what she had been told would be a life-long problem. I showed her energetic techniques to help her align her efforts more fully with her desire to be healthy, but she still would not do the exercises on her own.

In late September, I consulted my physician to review my condition and to obtain laboratory confirmation of the muscle testing results. Blood tests indicated elevated antibodies to Candida, including IgG, IgA, and IgM. She made the diagnosis of candidiasis and agreed that a yeast-free diet together with anti-Candida herbs was the best approach.

By early October, we continued to feel achy in the house and were increasingly sensitive to mold outside. We could no longer go for walks in the beautiful countryside. The deterioration in my health now limited my ability to appreciate that beauty. Often, I wished I had never heard of the Berkshires.

We continually looked for ways to lessen our mold sensitivities. I had bought an electronic homeopathic remedy machine from Jon Monroe which we now used to make our own autodetox remedies. I reasoned that if we knew which molds were bothering us most, I could use the remedy machine to make homeopathic remedies for them. To identify molds in the house I ordered mold plates. In mid-October, I exposed one plate each in eight different areas of the house and then returned them for processing. Patricia and I anxiously awaited these results.

Meantime, as the days of October passed, our frustrations mounted. We did not feel well in either place we were living. Patricia continued struggling to make her clothes wearable. Everything seemed unbearably difficult.

Upon returning to the Red House one Thursday, we were assailed by a perfume smell in our kitchen. Patricia recognized the scent worn by Marissa, our cat sitter, and found it was emanating from the kitchen table. Although we scrubbed the table repeatedly, we had to wait several days before we could eat at it again.

Patricia had been pleased with the way Marissa cared for her cats, but this one more chemical exposure was too much. It had been Patricia's experience in the past that when she approached people about the fact that their cologne or perfume made her ill, they were quite surprised and offended. Marissa was no exception. When Patricia explained her dilemma, Marissa said she understood, because she herself had allergies. Wishing Patricia luck in finding someone else to care for her cats, Marissa quickly and politely said good-bye. There seemed to be no room for negotiation around wearing perfume or not. Patricia's fear and shame over asking someone to do something they might not like to do kept her from pursuing the conversation further.

Over the next two weeks we made two important decisions. In light of how beneficial the Rochlitz work had been for us, I decided to try taking the training he was giving in November. A motel near him offered special arrangements for people with chemical sensitivities, including airing the room out for two days prior to arrival and using no toxic cleaners. The rooms had kitchens so that I would be able to cook my own food. We decided I could take three-days' worth of food with me and Patricia would come mid-week to replenish my supplies.

The second decision was for Patricia to go for MariEL healing as suggested to her when she consulted a spiritual advisor I had used in the past. Patricia asked her physician, massage therapist, and others what they knew about MariEL, but none had heard of it. After a lengthy search Patricia obtained the names of several MariEL practitioners in the Boston area. The only one with a current phone number was Adriana van Stralen who worked in Sharon, Massachusetts. When Patricia had spoken with Adriana two months earlier, she described MariEl as a gentle healing technique which facilitated the release of cellular memories from the body.

Patricia was intrigued by MariEl but at first resisted going. She felt the forty-minute trip from Watertown to Sharon would be too much on top of all the other driving we were doing. Finally, out of desperation she scheduled an appointment with Adriana on November seventh. During the week that followed, I planned to study with Steven Rochlitz in New York and Patricia would have time to herself in Great Barrington.

When the seventh came, Patricia felt sicker than she had in a long time. Her body hurt all over with flulike aching in her muscles and joints. Her head was very cloudy; she felt exhausted and had difficulty standing. Patricia attributed her symptoms to an elevated mold count caused by the rainy weather. Having myself had a body-work session in Concord that morning, I didn't feel like going anywhere; but when I saw how much trouble Patricia had just trying to stand up, I agreed to drive her to her appointment. She slept the whole way.

Adriana's directions led us easily to her house, a large, old colonial surrounded by woods. As I turned into the driveway, I awakened Patricia from her deep sleep. She was so unsteady that she needed my help to walk to the door. Adriana greeted us and expressed surprise that I had come. I told her I was Patricia's chauffeur for the day. She suggested things I could do while I waited, such as going to the nearby Audubon Sanctuary.

I took her advice and went for a walk. The light mist that had been falling on and off throughout the day had covered everything with moisture. As I followed the trail to the top of 500-foot-high Moose Hill, I smelled the odor of decaying leaves and noticed bright green mold on many trees. Muscle aching and fatigue made it impossible for me to take pleasure in the woods. How much had changed in a short time. Just two years earlier I had had an enjoyable visit to the same place at the same time of year. Now I had to stop my walk after a few minutes and returned to the house where I spent the next hour and a half in the foyer doing paperwork.

When Patricia finally came down the stairs, she was completely transformed. She appeared alert and refreshed with a healthy, rosy glow on her face. All her pain was gone. It astounded her that she felt both grounded and clear-headed with such a sense of peace. Patricia could remember very few times in her life when she felt so well. Only rare, fleeting moments of blissful meditation came close. She told me the experience was so wonderful that I had to try it. I was at a loss to explain the striking changes in her.

During the trip back to Watertown I learned more about what had happened. Adriana told Patricia it was unusual to start with a full MariEL treatment. Generally she worked with clients over time to prepare them. She made an exception in Patricia's case because of the specific recommendation Patricia received to have MariEL.

Patricia told me that as she lay on the massage table fully dressed, Adriana lightly touched her and then moved her hands above and away from her body. Adriana repeated these movements many times. Guided by Adriana, Patricia began breathing deeply and experienced deeper relaxation with each breath. She kept her eyes closed throughout most of the treatment and saw many colors and images. Particularly disturbing was an image she had seen before, perhaps in a dream, of a baby's body chopped into pieces but without any blood. This foreboding image aroused intense uneasiness. Patricia just wanted it to go away. Otherwise the session was extremely relaxing. Patricia was delighted by how she felt at the end of her session. Adriana told Patricia the process would continue for several days and she should rest, walk outside, lie on the ground, take hot baths, and use her breath to release any more pain that appeared.

The next afternoon we drove to Great Barrington. Patricia remained pain-free for three days. If any pain recurred, she remembered how she released it with her breath during the MariEL session and did so again. At times I complained of achiness caused by the mold outside. Patricia then felt guilty, because she felt wonderful and I did not. As we had done for months, I was vigilant to the effects of various smells in the house and discussed what needed to be done about them. Patricia noted that with each comment I made, a bit more of her joint and muscle pain returned. She became very annoyed with me but said nothing at the time about her feelings.

On Saturday morning, we awoke at four o'clock. While Patricia prepared food for me to take for the next three days, I loaded my car with the supplies, which I hoped would let me stay safely in the motel for a week. I packed a barrier cloth to put on the motel mattress, all-cotton sheets and blankets, a water filter, a special heater in case of cold weather, three air filters, an antimold device, two coolers full of food, and cookware. This carful of paraphenalia underscored how much I now needed to protect myself from the world.

At six-thirty I said good-bye to Patricia and left her to enjoy the remnants of her MariEL treatment. She appeared relieved to have a break from my comments about mold and chemical exposures, comments which now irritated her and made her feel separate from me.

I made better time than expected and checked into the motel before the seminar. My room was in a building set back from the road. As agreed, it had been aired out for forty-eight hours. In spite of this effort, I quickly developed symptoms, including nausea and muscle aching. Paneling on two walls and a mold smell inside and outside the room led me to question whether I could stay there.

Nevertheless, I unpacked and then went to class.

It was only a fifteen-minute drive to Steven's. The living room where Patricia and I had our consultations was now a crowded classroom. Seventeen professionals and lay people from across the United States and abroad attended the seminar. We learned a variety of muscle testing and energy-balancing techniques. Each time we learned a new technique, we practiced it with a partner. I found the material as fascinating as I had during our initial meeting. Here was an approach that worked with the body's inherent intelligence and self-corrective properties.

Even the class was not free of chemical exposures. When I smelled cologne, which increased my nausea and muscle tightness, I attempted to avoid the odor by moving to a corner of the room away from all but two other people. I tried focusing on the class and ignoring my symptoms, but it was no use. During a break I told Steven I was reacting to what someone was wearing. I requested he inform the others of the importance of avoiding scented products, because at least one person there had environmental illness. After he made an announcement to that effect, several other class members spoke about their own chemical sensitivities.

By the end of the first day, I felt energetic and clearheaded despite having been exposed to cologne and to mold outside. What we learned definitely helped. I decided to attend as many of the seven days of classes I had preregistered for as possible. I also concluded I could not stay at the motel because it was too moldy. The only way for me to go to the seminar would be to commute daily from Great Barrington. The distance roundtrip was approximately 180 miles and would take two hours each way. I wanted to do it; I would try.

After telephoning Patricia to let her know about this change in plans, I went to the motel to pick up my things. The trip along the winding country roads took longer at night. By the time I arrived back in Great Barrington at nine o'clock, my muscles ached from driving so much. Patricia was distressed by the disruption of her solitude but kept her feelings to herself. She told me she had spent most of the day outside, grounding the effects of her MariEL treatment. After showing her what we had learned in class, I went to sleep in order to wake up early the next day.

The next two days followed the same pattern. I woke at five o'clock, got ready, ate breakfast, drove two hours to New York, spent seven hours in class with an hour lunch break, drove two hours home, had dinner, and went to bed. By the fourth day this schedule had taken its toll. I felt tired and achy from too much driving and too little sleep. While the course material was informative and helpful, I did not know how I would complete the rest of the seminar at the same pace.

That day Donald, another participant, showed me a device that he had used to increase his energy. When he had mentioned it the day before, I asked him to bring the device so that I could try it. Its arrival could not have been more timely. The "Bio-Tron Projector" was a white cylinder approximately the size of a rural mailbox. It was made of hard plastic with a light bulb at one end and a Lucite panel at the other. When the light was turned on, its rays traveled the length of the cylinder and passed through the Lucite. The Bio-Tron Projector had been invented by the late Dan Roehm, a retired physician who marketed it as an educational device.

The user of the Bio-Tron Projector sits or lies in its beam. According to the late Dr. Roehm in his pamphlet, "Introducing the Biotron Era," the device works by concentrating biotrons and projecting them to the user. He described the biotron as "a fundamental energizing particle of the universe" and estimated biotrons from the sun and stars already account for one-third of our energy. He claimed his device effectively increased the amount of biotrons available to the body.

Donald put the Bio-Tron Projector on the floor next to me and turned it on. In less than five seconds I felt a surge of energy inside and insisted he turn it off. While many people used the device for up to eight hours per day, clearly I could not. Feeling dizzy and nauseous, I went outside to recover from this initial contact. The fresh air helped, but I needed to rest. I went to sit in my car for a few moments and was startled when I woke up forty-five minutes later. The afternoon session had already begun. Quickly collecting myself, I returned to class. After I sat down, I realized I felt more energized and my muscles were more relaxed as if a layer of symptoms had been lifted.

The Bio-Tron Projector appeared to have helped, but how could I use it in a way that did not put me to sleep? Working with muscle testing, I determined the optimal length of time for me to be in its beam, and the optimal distance. At first the testing indicated one hour at a distance of twenty feet. Using these parameters, I positioned the Bio-Tron Projector so that I received its effects while sitting in class. I then experienced the benefits of greater energy and muscle relaxation without feeling exhausted.

After muscle testing indicated using the Bio-Tron Projector more that day would be helpful, Donald let me borrow it for the night. When I returned home, I told Patricia about the device, and, of course, she wanted to try it too. Muscle testing indicated she should use it for only ten minutes. She also experienced benefits, including feelings of lightness and energy in her body.

The next morning I woke up spontaneously at four o'clock, feeling alert and energized. I was so excited I shook Patricia and exclaimed that the Bio-Tron Projector really worked! Before leaving, I called to order one and requested that it be sent as soon as possible. That morning I returned Donald's machine to him, but for the rest of the seminar he brought it each day and let me use it during class. Between doing the energy balancing exercises we learned and using the Bio-Tron Projector, I completed all seven days of the seminar for which I had preregistered. I continued to have reactions at times but generally tolerated them better than before.

By Friday afternoon, I had come to appreciate Steven as an excellent teacher who integrated the areas of energy-balancing, kinesiology, nutrition, and ecology. Reflecting on all I had learned, I considered taking the course "Advanced Ecology and Meta-Integration," which was being taught the next two days. When Patricia and I discussed the seminar that evening, she voiced concern that I was overextending myself. I argued that Steven's material had helped us more than anything else thus far. I wanted to take advantage of the opportunity to learn more. Finally, I decided to go.

Over the week I had attended the seminar, Patricia's frustration had escalated. The benefits of the MariEL treatment had left her. After being symptom-free for three days, she was depressed by the gradual return of muscle aching, joint pain, nausea, and other symptoms. A major annoyance was her inability to salvage her paint-contaminated clothing despite countless washings. At her wit's end, she had been considering the recommendation of an expert on dealing with chemicals that she ozone the clothing to neutralize any remaining paint. Just mentioning the ozone machine made me cringe because of all the grief it had caused us. Patricia saw it as her only hope to have clothes to wear.

For me, Saturday and Sunday sped by. When the class ended late Sunday afternoon, I felt thoroughly saturated with this new material and was eager to share it with Patricia. I said good-bye to my classmates and hurried back to Great Barrington. Driving up the steep hill to the Red House, I savored feelings of accomplishment. I had completed nine days of the seminar in spite of many obstacles. These feelings ended abruptly as I turned into the driveway.

I was stunned to see Patricia walking around the yard in a daze, her clothing strewn everywhere. As I rushed over to find out what had happened, noxious odors assaulted me. I had to shake her by the shoulders to get her to talk coherently. She told me she had followed suggested guidelines for ozoning her clothing by putting several items into a large wardrobe box outside and then turning the ozone machine on for fifteen minutes. She broke into tears as she said that she had been airing many items for several hours and still the strong chemical smell would not go away.

Upon hearing what Patricia had done, my anxiety level skyrocketed. Rather than improving the situation, she had made things much worse. Now her clothing reeked of chemicals, and there was danger those strong smells would contaminate the rest of the house.

# CHAPTER EIGHT

# Tortuous Transition

Although we constantly focused on avoiding chemicals, we were again faced with a major exposure. By ozoning her clothing all together Patricia inadvertently created a chemical soup, which then contaminated everything she was working on. Her goal had been to eliminate lingering traces of paint fumes. Instead, she was left with clothing that smelled of paint, dry cleaning fluid, and other unidentified substances. This latest episode in her clothes saga was one more intensification in our war with environmental illness. It also marked the beginning of the end. Over the next month our suffering would be magnified to the extent that we could not continue to live as we had. Fortunately, we would be guided to a way out.

When Patricia tried on the ozoned clothing, the reality of this latest fiasco sank in. Whatever she wore worsened her symptoms. Although she had not been able to wear her paint-tainted clothes, she had clung to the hope of making them wearable. Now that possibility was lost; she had ruined all her clothes. She had no money for new ones and could not have tolerated their chemicals anyway. We stored the casualties of this latest battle in plastic bags in the basement.

The next day I called the company where I had bought the ozone machine to ask their suggestions. They said the ozoning should have been done one garment at a time for brief intervals with frequent airing. Upon hearing about the damage to all of Patricia's clothing they offered a special recipe used to remove chemicals when everything else had failed. It involved washing and soaking the clothing with various substances. One treatment took a day or more, but at least it was something else we could try.

I immediately drove to the local supermarket and bought four gallons of vinegar, a large box of powdered milk, and all the baking soda they had. I tried the new washing recipe on an organic cotton sweat shirt, which Patricia had bought several months earlier. When the process was done, the shirt smelled of vinegar and milk so we decided to leave those steps out. Patricia was still unable to wear it without developing headaches and nausea. Although the shirt was made from organic cotton, the cotton had been grown with organic pesticides, and apparently Patricia was reacting to them.

Patricia coped with these latest developments in several ways. At times she lapsed into panicked sobbing. At others she raged in anger about the unfairness of all she had been through and her failure to get well even with all her efforts. There was a daily struggle just to get a piece of clothing she could wear. Frequently, she wore my clothes to work. Most of the time she cooked. That was one area where she felt some sense of control while the rest of her life was falling apart.

Rather than our problems lessening, they grew. When we returned to the Red House the next Friday, I was surprised to smell Patricia's ozoned clothes as I entered the front door. I wondered where the smell was coming from, because we kept them in the basement. The answer was right in front of me. They were in a laundry basket next to the cellar door. We had been so disoriented when we last went to Boston that we left her clothes out. I was dismayed to discover that my clothing, which was on a table nearby to keep it free of odors, now smelled like Patricia's. When I tried a shirt on, I developed muscle aching, nausea, and dizziness. I could not wear it. As a result of our mistake most of my wardrobe was contaminated. I was left with only what I carried between Great Barrington and Watertown in a suitcase. I added my toxic clothes to the other belongings in the basement, to be salvaged.

The next time we went to Watertown we discovered more trouble. As soon as we entered the apartment, we smelled natural gas.

The apartment's heat was forced hot air by natural gas which we had not used in over a year. In fact, we had covered the ceiling heating vents with denny foil to prevent gas fumes from entering the apartment. Now we urgently needed to find out where the smell was coming from to avoid an explosion of leaking gas. Removing the foil failed to reveal the source of the smell, so I called the gas company and arranged for an emergency inspection. The technician used his detection device and found no evidence of a leak. He said he smelled no gas and assured us it was safe. We had our doubts but proceeded with caution in the apartment.

I became aware that week of my extreme sensitivity to the smell of natural gas elsewhere as well. Whenever the gas heat in my office came on I developed motor incoordination, disorientation, fatigue, and muscle aching. It had been enough of a struggle to work even with my chemical sensitivities, but I now faced this new obstacle. I coped by having the heating vent in my office disconnected and using an electric heater. Then I felt better in the office but developed symptoms when I went out into the hall. My awareness of the gas fumes from the kitchen stove two doors down from me was so acute that I often rushed out to see if there were a gas leak. It was merely the gas pilot light or someone using the stove.

When we returned to the Watertown apartment on the last Monday in November, we again smelled the strong odor of natural gas. I called the gas company to arrange for another emergency inspection. This time the technician was a woman who listened carefully to our concerns. She used her most sensitive measuring devices and detected nothing. After we told her we still smelled gas, she went down to the basement three floors below where she turned off the gas line to my apartment. Then we no longer smelled gas and our gas-related symptoms in the apartment ceased. It seemed we were more sensitive than the most delicate measuring instruments.

Patricia and I began reacting to gas heat in the natural foods grocery store where we had shopped for years without difficulty. Nausea, dizziness, and disorientation made it hard not only to focus on what we wanted to buy but also just to move around the store. Our panic escalated further. We worried our increased sensitivity meant we were getting sicker and our lives would become even more restricted. We were completely bewildered. We no longer knew what to think, what to do, or where to turn.

The next trip to Great Barrington provided some direction. In the mailbox were the results of the mold plates which I had exposed in eight different parts of the house. The plates each grew from four to eight different kinds of mold with colony counts as high as fifty-eight. (Seven types of mold, or over eight colony counts total per plate, indicates the need for serious environmental controls.) These results signaled major mold infestation throughout the whole house. We had known there was a mold problem, but the extent of the contamination suggested we had been fighting a losing battle. Constant exposure to that much mold had been an ongoing insult to our immune systems. No wonder our unceasing efforts had failed to lead to recovery.

We next considered what to do about living in that much toxicity. My first response was to figure out how to correct it. After much discussion, we decided the amount of mold combined with our heightened sensitivity meant we could no longer live there. If we wanted to get better, we had to move from the living hell of a place which was supposed to help us get well.

Just thinking about leaving the moldy house with the many rooms we could not use brought feelings of relief, but there were problems too. How would we get out of the lease? Where would we move? Where would we do laundry? How would we get well?

The lease question was answered fairly easily. I called Jacob and informed him of the mold plate results. He was concerned both about our health and about his house. When I told him that the level of mold contamination combined with our deteriorated health meant we had to move, he agreed to negotiate early termination of our lease. We eventually settled on April fifteenth. Patricia and I surmised he would happy to be rid of us.

To answer our questions about what to do next and how to get better, we turned to an old friend for advice. Over the years I had consulted "Michael" through various channels on many occasions. He is an entity, or collection of souls, who previously lived on Earth many times. After completing their learning here, these souls joined together to form their entity, which now offers assistance from the mid-causal plane. Michael's message is one of unconditional acceptance of self and others. His teachings describe the ways the individual essence, or soul, takes on different personalities through many lifetimes to learn various lessons. I had found his information refreshing and insightful.

I initially had reservations about channeling, but experiences with Michael had cleared my doubts. He offered a valuable per-spective on the world. I especially appreciated the way he always reminded me to take nothing that he said for granted and encour-aged me to validate it with the truth within myself. I called Mary Jonaitis, the channel with whom I had worked recently, and arranged for two one-hour readings with Michael over the phone.

When Saturday December fourteenth came, we hoped Michael would offer a new point of view, a way out of the black hole we were collapsing into. Patricia went first in the early afternoon. I heard her laughing and wondered what was so funny. At the end of the hour I impatiently asked what Michael had said. She replied that, according to him, we had created our illness. I became so angry that I wanted to cancel my session, and I demanded to know how he could say such a thing. I insisted I had a physical illness and my reactions were caused by dysfunction of my immune system. Patricia seemed comfortable with Michael's comments and even somewhat amused. She recalled screaming at me months earlier that in all her years with environmental illness, her life had never been so bizarre and out of control. Michael's explanation offered her the possibility of freedom to create a different reality.

By five o'clock my anger had subsided enough for me to talk with Michael. When I asked about the status of my health, he replied that my nervous system was stronger than a year ago with a more consistent pattern of vibration. He stated that all immune system disorders are related to the health of the nervous system/spiritual channel. He added that the first transformation of the physical can be made at the level of the nervous system. When I asked about my heightened sensitivities to chemicals, Michael said that my sensitivities had to do with the belief that something could harm me or the belief that there was something to which I was sensitive. He advised me not to be concerned about the sensitivities persisting because they would fade as I eliminated the belief forms.

Barely able to control the anger I felt at being told my illness was caused by my beliefs, I said that from his comments, belief forms seemed critical in creating illness. Michael responded that belief is critical for everyone living on the physical plane. When the belief factor is engaged, a number of treatments can help at the physical level. Those same treatments will not work if the belief factor is not dealt with. Michael added that the factor of belief is important for everything in life. Learning is achieved in different ways. Some choose an illness, some an accident, some a bad marriage, and some a constant struggle with money. When there is struggle at any level, there is a sense of something having power over the being. The being gives this "something" the power to take over.

I asked about the best way to work with the belief factor. Michael said the best approach would be conscious choosing, which was part of the work of Arnold Mindell, Barry Kaufman, Deepak Chopra, and others. He especially recommended Chopra's work which, he said, emphasizes that matter does not exist except for that which is created. Chopra presents an interweaving of modern physics and the Ayurvedic view in a readily available style.

The role of belief in illness seemed interesting, theoretically, but I wanted to know how it applied to me. I reviewed my eighteen months with environmental illness and asked how my beliefs were related to my initial symptoms and to life in the Red House, which continued to get progressively worse. Michael said that the house had been playing a game with us, the game of "what reality can we create here?" He said this game grew out of a pattern of thoughts I was unconsciously holding, based on an underlying belief that something external could determine how I chose to create my life. He added that you create whatever you put your conscious attention on. By thinking about what caused a certain symptom, you would eventually find many causes for that symptom as well as many other symptoms, because the mind is giving a lot of attention to symptoms, responses, and reactions.

I protested I would be very happy to be free of the symptoms which had been tormenting me. Michael answered certainly, consciously, I would choose to let go of my illness, but he emphasized that at an unconscious level I did not believe in my true freedom to create physical reality. As a result, creating physical reality in accordance with my desires was not yet available to me.

Michael explained further how unconsciously held beliefs affect one's reality. He compared beliefs to an armature, the framework used by sculptors to form a figure from plastic material. Since the material is too soft to stand on its own, it is molded over the armature, which gives it support. Michael said beliefs at a deep level serve as a kind of armature over which life experiences are layered. For me the belief that something outside of myself determined my experience served as the framework over which energy and, subsequently, matter were layered to create my experiences of that belief.

Michael said that in order for me to heal myself I had to break down the skeleton of who I was at a spiritual, mental, and emotional level and create a new one. He described this breaking-down process as involving going around and around trying to find the truth of how to find my own freedom. In the process of trying very hard to find my freedom, I was coming into a state of giving up or of not knowing which way to go next and also to a state of boredom with the process of constantly having to deal with one stupid detail after another. The absurd quantity of details made them seem stupid. Eventually, a kind of boredom would ensue, a kind of breaking down of the mind's interest in dealing with all of this. I would reach the point that room would be made for a new paradigm of sight or vision from which I could begin to build a new reality. Michael added, in other words this was a death process. He then asked for my comments.

I said I *felt* like I was dying. Michael responded that parts of me should die, the parts that held the forms of perceptions or beliefs which I no longer needed. He reminded me that even before I developed environmental illness he had told me people create everything. He said, again, that everybody is making up everything and there is nothing but making it up. He emphasized the importance of understanding that it does not have to take a long time to shift beliefs once there is complete willingness to do so.

Michael then spoke about the unique aspects of environmental illness. He said it takes a very complicated mind to live the reality of environmental illness. Environmental illness is a truly creative act in the sense that there is more complexity to it all the time. That ever-increasing complexity generates great frustration and irritation. Michael commented that I had an active, complicated mind which was very fertile. The mind could be a powerful creative tool or a powerful destructive tool depending on the armature I was holding to build on.

I told him what he said was of great interest, but I wanted to know what he recommended as a next step to help us escape this living nightmare of environmental illness. Michael suggested we begin to experience our reactions as a witness or an observer. We could thereby begin to let go of our judgments, labeling this as "good" and that as "bad." He said this practice would provide some of the first stepping stones out of the depths of this illness.

He elaborated on how this process would work. In observing, or witnessing, we could start to put less meaning into our reactions. He said that we had invested a lot of meaning in them, but when you get down to basic reality, nothing has more meaning than anything else. Life has no meaning, because it is essentially a big playground, a big art studio in which everything is being created and invested with meaning for the purpose of learning through experience. The more meaning you put into an experience, the more real it becomes. The less meaning you put into it, the less real and the less compelling it becomes. Then you can drop it.

Michael said environmental illness fosters the process of investing things and experiences with meaning. When someone is sensitive, more and more things start to support that view of the world. This is safe, that is unsafe. Some will start to think that maybe they will be okay if they stay away from what is unsafe. The problem is there is no such thing. It is all just world. He added that the only way to remove the power of the meanings of the unsafe parts of the world is to stand back and observe, to let at least one part of yourself stand back and watch, not judging this is safe, that is unsafe, this is bad and that is good.

I was having a hard time absorbing everything Michael was saying but wanted to take something immediately applicable away from the session. I asked what we should do when symptoms of a reaction came on. He said observe, or, if you have a way to work with the symptoms for the moment, do that. But do not feel what you do will save your life and do not put meaning into it, because what works for one person one day may not work for another the next. Similarly, with problems such as mold, Michael said the difficulties persisted because we had not let go of that physical reality. He advised working with the mold as needed but without giving it excess meaning.

I then asked Michael's assessment of the kinesiology I had been using with Patricia. He said it allowed her to tune into messages her consciousness wanted to give her. Messages from the inner self may come through thoughts, feelings, or the physical body. When more subtle messages are not being listened to, the body has to get more and more extreme in the messages it gives. The kinesiology sessions had brought Patricia's awareness to those parts of herself which were trying to communicate with her. Her conscious mind could then begin to bring the messages through more directly, thereby taking her body off the hook. Michael recommended I have Patricia use kinesiology with me to discover when I had lost the sense of being free to choose my life.

At that point Michael switched topics. He said another approach to healing is to work on finding the bliss inside yourself at all times no matter what the situation may be, no matter how hellish your life may be. Finding this bliss within, which he termed "the natural happiness" available to each human no matter what, recreates a natural, authentic state. Otherwise there is a tendency to be constantly looking for security or safety in the outer world where it does not exist.

As the end of the hour neared, I asked Michael if I created everything in my life, why had I created this illness which so devastated me. He replied that the illness was a shamanic experience from which I could draw to myself enormous power as a healer. While much of what Michael said that day aggravated me, these words piqued my interest. Perhaps there was a purpose in all the pain and suffering we had been going through. In the months ahead I would return to his words for solace when I reached points where I felt unable to continue on.

Michael closed our session by reminding me it is all dream and I am a dreamer dreaming up the dream. He asked me to think about how I wanted that dream to be and said this would help me determine it. He sent me love and asked me to accept the beautiful abundance of the universe, the support and love which were there for me. He offered hope that I would soon be able to come through this time of tribulation and experience my full freedom and joyful vitality every day. He offered his support on what he described as "this beautiful path."

As I put the phone down, my head was spinning. There was a sinking feeling in my stomach. What was it Michael had said? Had I created this illness which was destroying my life? I knew I had a physical problem. My immune system was broken, and I was sensitive to nearly everything. Taken on their own terms, Michael's comments made sense, but how did they apply to us? If this illness were our creation, were we to blame for all the suffering we had been through? Most importantly, would changing our beliefs lead to improved health? The next eighteen months would answer this last question.

Patricia and I discussed our sessions at length. I was intrigued by the reference to my illness as a shamanic experience, but the idea that I had created it still infuriated me. Patricia, who had undergone more of the breaking-down process, readily embraced Michael's explanation. Since nothing else had produced dramatic and sustained improvement, we decided to try his suggestions.

We began by experimenting with various forms of meditation to see which ones would allow us to experience the silent witness even in the midst of reactions. Although I had meditated daily for more than twenty years, no practice had been as challenging as this effort to return to health. We found that mantra meditation, involving focusing on a sound, and meditation on counting the breath both had the effect we wanted. When we put them into action, we were pleased by the results.

Warm, rainy weather two days later produced high mold levels outside. When it was that moldy, I typically felt heavy and sluggish and my muscles ached. By doing mantra meditation in the morning and as needed throughout the day, I was able to remain free of mold symptoms. It rained again the following day, and Patricia decided to try this technique herself. She had worked only briefly with meditation in the past. This time she persisted. Her muscles ached much less than usual for a rainy day. She also stayed alert instead of collapsing at the late afternoon peak mold time.

Encouraged by our initial success, we looked for other occasions to try to alter our reactions. Driving to my office the following day offered such an opportunity. When I discovered my car's air filter was not working, I panicked and became angry; the filter allowed me to drive safely in traffic. Without it exhaust fumes invaded my car causing muscle aching, nausea, and irritability. This time when I began to feel sick, I meditated on a mantra. An inner voice said "try using this as an opportunity to reprogram your reactions to the exhaust." The combination of meditation and reprogramming led to a marked reduction in my symptoms. Any remaining ones were cleared by doing meta-integration exercises, advanced energy-balancing techniques developed by Steven Rochlitz, after I reached my office.

While these experiments with meditation demonstrated the possibility of lessening our symptoms through shifting our consciousness, there were limitations. To achieve maximum benefit we had to remember to do the meditations constantly throughout the day. Even then not all sensitivities went away. Although Patricia was more receptive to Michael's suggestions, she had greater difficulty putting them into action. The degree of her sensitivities together with extreme fatigue made it hard for her to think clearly, let alone meditate.

Michael also recommended conscious choosing as a way to health, including the work of Deepak Chopra. When we listened to Chopra's tape set, *Magical Mind Magical Body*, we were spurred on by his comments. He described quantum physics understanding of the human being as paralleling that of Ayurveda, ancient India's science of life.

Chopra said that while western medicine tends to focus on the body as the ultimate reality, quantum physics views the body as predominantly empty space. He emphasized that this space is not an empty void but a fullness of information and intelligence which interacts with itself to produce the mind and the body. He summarized by saying that rather than being a body which has learned to think, we are intelligence which has learned to create a body. We humans continually create our body. The problem is we keep creating it the same way over and over. Chopra said that by aligning more fully with our inner intelligence we can learn to create health even when there has been serious illness, such as cancer or heart disease. We wondered whether a similar approach would work for environmental illness.

While we followed up on Michael's recommendations, we continued making the necessary adjustments to move out of Great Barrington. We quit our jobs in western Massachusetts. We moved whatever we would need in the immediate future to the Watertown apartment, where the back bedroom served as our decontamination chamber. It soon was filled with items we wanted to use but which were too toxic to bring into the rest of the apartment.

We would have been happy never to go back to the Red House, but it was the one safe place we had to do laundry. We tried the washer in the apartment building, but residue from other peoples' detergents tainted our things with odors that made us sick. It was particularly frustrating to have used that washer for years without difficulty and now to have to drive two and a half hours for a washing machine that was safe for us.

There even were laundry problems in Great Barrington. The washer seemed all right, but Patricia began noticing the faint smell of perfumed, fabric softener squares on items as they came out of the dryer. After attempts to clean up the landlord's old dryer failed, I bought a new one. Amidst our constant stress and mental confusion we failed to consider the chemicals on the new dryer which had to be dealt with before we could safely use it. For days we washed the dryer drum with Super Clean and alternately turned it on and aired it to outgas its chemicals. When the dryer was finally ready, we used it to dry our laundry as well as in ongoing efforts to detoxify contaminated clothing and to make new clothes wearable.

On our drives back and forth across the state, we noticed a phenomenon we had not observed before. Often the window next to me in the car fogged up. We tried unsuccessfully to come up with a rational explanation. Finally, we decided it indicated energy I was releasing. Patricia's window fogged up too but not so dramatically. Whenever we noticed the window fogging, we laughed. It felt like we had not laughed in a long time.

We celebrated Christmas 1991 by staying in eastern Massachusetts for a week. It was a welcome respite from hours of driving and the moldy house. During that time we reflected on the unbelievable series of events we had been through as a result of environmental illness and anticipated what lay ahead.

We both were much more sensitive than when we joined forces to try to get better. Our experiments with energetically oriented approaches like the Rochlitz exercises and MariEL clearly demonstrated the possibility of improvement, but we needed to find some way to sustain it. Our daily routine was so complicated and demanding that we had been unable to incorporate silent witnessing into our daily lives. From Michael's perspective, we were in the midst of a deep healing, part of a transition to greater health. From our perspective, we were struggling to fight our way out of quicksand.

As we looked to 1992, we considered where to direct our efforts. What would help us truly heal ourselves? Others we knew with environmental illness were either steadily deteriorating or giving their all to maintain a dysfunctional status quo. In order to become well we would have to do something radically different.

# PART III

# Transformation

January 1992—July 1993

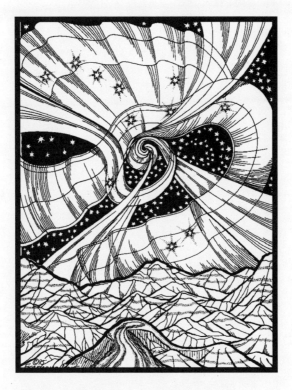

"The problems we have created at one
level cannot be solved at that level but
only by moving to another level."

*Albert Einstein*

# CHAPTER NINE

# Going Within

We began 1992 by resolving to study the inner dimensions of environmental illness. We committed ourselves to discovering what role thoughts, feelings, and spirit had played in our becoming sick and could play in our recovery. There were no books related to environmental illness on this subject. We were on our own. We had no idea what we were getting into.

On January fourth we unwittingly pursued our goal by attending an all-day seminar at the Greenwood House in Sharon, where Adriana and several other practitioners of the healing arts resided. Pat Balzer, a woman from Maine, was coming to give a talk on the 11:11, which Adriana described as an energetic doorway that offered the potential for humanity to evolve to a higher state of consciousness. This was to be one of a series of events that began on December 31, 1986, and would continue over a twenty-five-year period.

I had felt a strong urge to participate in the second event, known as the Harmonic Convergence, which occurred on August 16 and 17, 1987. In fact, I had celebrated it twice on the same day, first in Hong Kong, then in Hawaii after crossing the International Dateline.

I had been excited to be part of this gathering of people of like minds around the globe, who had the intention to open to a wave of higher consciousness that would change the world as we know it. I knew I wanted to go to the talk on the 11:11.

Although attending a public event continued to be a challenge for us because of our reactions to the personal-care products worn by others, Adriana's enthusiastic endorsement of Pat, combined with our new willingness to experiment with ways to overcome reactions, led to our decision to go. When we arrived, the large living room was already filled with more than thirty people seated in a circle. As we squeezed into a corner, I said I hoped there would be no harmful smells near us. Patricia told me not to worry, that we would be fine. She reminded me that we always felt better at the Greenwood House.

Pat and her husband, Paul, arrived half an hour later. Snow had slowed their three-hour drive from Maine. Pat is a big woman with light brown hair and blue eyes whose presence emanates both gentleness and power. As she entered the room and sat down, I had an awareness of the enormous significance of this gathering. I reflected how dramatically my life had changed since the Harmonic Convergence and wondered what the 11:11 would bring.

Pat began by saying that she was a channel and briefly explained what that was like. Then she talked about Vywamus (pronounced Vie-*waa*-mus), the being she channeled. She described him as a great teacher who has a deep connection to humanity and to the Earth. She said he was here to assist us in the transformation that was now in progress. She emphasized that his focus when he came through her was to assist people in overcoming self-imposed limitations and to bring to their attention those areas of self which they have judged deeply, denied, and placed outside of their conscious awareness.

When she began to channel, immediately the room felt different. Vywamus' energy was intense and probing. I found it difficult to understand his words, but I was fascinated by what he had to say.

Vywamus said that for years the Earth had been permeated by judgment, which he defined as an energy that separates. He described the 11:11 as the union of two markedly different energies. On a cosmic level it was a union between the usual human framework of experiencing things and another framework which was familiar but had been pushed away by peoples' judgments. He said the energy which was coming to the Earth for this union was energy from which the Earth had been born. This process that the Earth and humanity were embarking on had the potential to bring about a much-needed completion of the understanding of the human body. Up to this point, judgments people hold have prevented humanity from gaining this understanding. He noted that people have particularly strong judgments about the physical and emotional bodies. He predicted that as this incoming energy intensified, judgment would also increase.

To help us grasp what he was talking about, Vywamus drew two large circles on the board. He said that Earth originated in one Source but had ended up in another. Life in this second Source, where we have lived, has centered around there being a boss and everyone's energies supporting that boss. The first Source, whose energies were increasing in intensity and from which the Earth originated, says there is a room full of cocreators, there is no one boss. As a result of the discrepancy between the Source people have been living under and the Source from which the Earth was made, humans have created structures that are out of alignment with the inherent flow of Earth energy.

According to Vywamus, the Earth's Original Source had been approaching the present Source for some time. They first touched at the etheric level two thousand years ago. Only later did we come to understand that Source referred to God or Universal Conciousness, that the meeting at the etheric level manifested on Earth as Jesus Christ, and that what he referred to as the Earth's Original Source is the Goddess Energy. He predicted the merging of these two sources would result in the creation of a new humanity, one fully integrating mind, body, spirit, and emotions.

The 11:11 would mark the opening of lines of energy flow from the Earth's Original Source into the Earth. This merging would catalyze many changes—each person becoming more in touch with who he or she is. Reflectivity would increase. Vywamus defined reflectivity as the process by which life mirrors back to someone unrecognized thoughts, emotions, and beliefs they are holding. For example, if individuals carry unexpressed rage inside, their bodies may manifest it through an angry, red rash or they may meet one angry person after another until they recognize their own rage. He recommended that as we had various images reflected back to us we approach ourselves in a loving way.

Vywamus elaborated on changes which would occur as a result of the 11:11. He said that while in the past unresolved thoughts or feelings were often pushed into the physical body, the physical body would no longer accept them. Mental and emotional conflicts would have to be resolved in their own right. Another change would be in the way people would love themselves. He noted that people often try to love themselves through loving others. Now people would be required to be fully who they are and to love themselves directly.

Vywamus' words resonated deeply within me. Although I comprehended only a fraction of what he said, I sensed he could help with my healing. When the seminar was over, I thanked Pat for her talk and asked for references on the ways the body reflects messages through various symptoms. She recommended Louise Hays' book, *You Can Heal Your Life.* When I expressed interest in talking with Vywamus about my illness, she scheduled a phone consultation to take place four days later. Patricia made an appointment too.

While we waited for our sessions with Vywamus, we continued to cope with the seemingly endless chemical exposures which constantly emerged in new and unexpected ways. At work on Monday morning when I entered the men's room, the muscles of my back and neck went into intense spasms and I became short of breath. I identified the source of this latest reaction as a blue disinfectant that had been placed in the toilet over the weekend. Every time the toilet was flushed, more chemicals were released. After enduring the reactions twice, I took corrective action. Donning rubber gloves and a charcoal mask, I removed the disinfectant container and put it in the janitor's closet and hoped that would end the problem.

When Wednesday evening finally came, I was eager to hear what Vywamus had to say about my illness and how to overcome it. I soon discovered his answers were quite different from what one might expect.

Vywamus greeted me and asked what I wanted to talk about. I described my illness to him and asked for any insights he could give me. He responded by saying I was composed of more than I wanted to think I was. He saw me as reluctant to recognize all of who I was. I preferred the intellect that I used to quantify and qualify myself and that, in fact, was part of the cause of my reactions. He said my healing would involve surrendering to inner parts of myself and experiencing my body and feelings in ways to which I was not accustomed. He acknowledged I had pursued a spiritual quest but said I had limited it to the realms of the mind and spirit where I enjoyed the fast-paced movement and sense of freedom. I had avoided the slower-paced realms of the body and emotions. This notion that somehow I had been cutting myself off from parts of myself was totally foreign to me.

Vywamus asked how I felt when I was having an allergic reaction. I said it varied; but often my thinking became confused, my muscles became tight, and it was hard for me to move. Vywamus viewed the slowing down and confusion I experienced as beneficial effects of my environmental illness, because I was forced to sit and feel parts of myself where I normally was not present. He added that when I was slowed down, I fought against it and tried to speed up again, rather than giving myself permission to experience the slowing down as a normal and essential part of the process—the process of connecting to the inside of myself. He said there was almost an allergic reaction to the inner parts of my self.

Vywamus astounded me by saying I had invoked my illness. He said the answer to my prayers and intentions to fulfill my purpose required that all of me be present including parts which I had neglected. Because of my tendency to avoid accepting unconditionally certain aspects of my self, I had created situations in which I was locked into experiencing those very aspects. The more I resisted this process, the more I took on projects that took me outside of myself, the more intensified my symptoms became to put me back inside. He said I merely needed to sit down and surrender to this process, which was going to put me in touch with all of who I was.

Vywamus said opening to areas within myself which I had avoided required a clearing of deeply ingrained patterns. He facilitated the beginning of this clearing through a powerful meditation. First, he had me visualize a golden tube of light going down into the Earth and spinning around me. He then verbally identified some of my patterns and told me to release them into the golden tube. For example, he said, "Letting go of the need to experience constriction, loss of life, health, and enjoyment as I seek to understand and connect with the physical and emotional aspects of who I am now." As I did the meditation, I sensed strong energy shifts throughout my body.

According to Vywamus, I feared being fully present in my body and emotions and was angry about having to deal with the physical-emotional parts of myself. He said I did not think I should have to experience anything emotional or physical. In addition, I feared that if I did, I would lose all the joy I had ever had, I would suffocate, I would die. He said fear associated with this convoluted flow was layered deep into my belief structure.

My emotional and physical bodies had been attempting to integrate the energy which had been flowing increasingly to the Earth in the past two years. They now worried that if they truly embraced that energy, my mental and spiritual bodies would leave them. As a result my emotional and physical bodies were resisting fully embracing the energy which was coming in, even though it was truly nourishing to them.

Vywamus next pointed out that in the past as I had stored conflicts in my body, I had become numb to the pain involved. The clearing process would entail experiencing it. Since I was reluctant to touch this emotional pain, I literally put it through the physical structure. He added that by ignoring the pain initially as I stored the conflicts in my physical body I had pushed the energy in very tightly. In denying the associated distress by saying this is not real, this

is not spiritual, this is not mental, this is not in my reality, I had sub-
jected my emotional and physical bodies to more abuse than if I had
let myself feel the pain.

Vywamus called my environmental illness a drastic approach to
clearing out areas that did not truly support me. He asked me to
consider cleaning out the basement of the Red House as symbolic
of attempts to clear out lower parts of my self. As I cleared out the
basement, I was impacted physically. As the stuckness inside me
started to move, it did not feel good. The clearing in me had been
stimulated by the energy coming to the Earth. He said such a drastic approach had been necessary because it was critical for the
clearing to be done now. He said it was as if I decided to clean my
basement out after it had been flooded, rather than fixing the holes
when the first puddles showed up.

Feeling beaten down by Vywamus' comments, I asked what
could be done about the problems he described. He replied that first
of all I should stop blaming my body for being allergic. The body
was simply expressing to me what I had pushed outside of myself.
I had chosen to push various conflicts and issues outside myself,
and my body was simply mirroring them back to me. He said in my
own way I really did not like being on the Earth. For me it was too
slow, I saw no purpose in it, no refinement, and found it very
annoying. He kept pounding away at his point, saying I really did
not want to be here. I would rather sit in my mind and journey in
my mind.

He went on to say the fact was I was here, but I was playing the
game that I did not want to be here and refusing to recognize I was
here. When I did recognize I was here, all I wanted to do was rage
about it. The physical-emotional body which brought me here
ended up getting pushed far away, and all I did was get angrier at
it. He said in the past I could engage in denial about this and it
would be buffered so that I did not see it. He likened it to the alco-
holic who drinks for twenty years and the family goes along with it
and all of a sudden they become annoyed. My physical and emotional bodies would no longer accept the denial.

He emphasized that I had chosen this situation. I was the one invoking wholeness, I was the one who wanted to discover who I was, I was the one who had been pulling light into my body through meditation. These intentions and actions had created movement inside of me. I had invoked the process, and now I was going through it. By the time I was finished I would have greater understanding of who I was, how I could affect myself, and what I did to show myself things I resisted owning.

Vywamus bombarded me with one comment after another about aspects of myself I had been avoiding. He told me I had sat for lifetimes on mountain tops praying to be taken away and had spent lifetimes in monasteries meditating to purify myself in order to leave my body. He said all those efforts had not worked, and I had come back to "get it." Coming back to get my body meant I would have to deal with all the issues I had when I tried to leave it behind. That was part of what I was going through now.

He said I approached my body from a mental perspective, always with the attitude that the mind was superior to the body. In doing so I neither honored nor blessed the body. I failed to experience the body in its own right. I needed to learn to honor and bless everything I had created from a soul level. I had created the present opportunity for me to be in a situation where I could restructure the mental box in which I had imprisoned my body. Vywamus said then I would honor the physical when it was flowing.

He commented that in the past I had approached my body like a mechanical machine, never seeing the glory of God in it, never really looking at it as something miraculous. He described my illness as a mental perspective layered over my physical body in a way that did not honor my body's wholeness. Consequently, my body could not express its wholeness back to me. It could only express what I had decided it was. Vywamus encouraged me to focus on loving and appreciating my body. He added that in the process I should give myself permission to go beyond the attitude that the physical body was just a pain in the butt.

Vywamus then gave me affirmations to work with for two

weeks. He suggested I think of them like stones dropped into the lake of my consciousness, rippling outward in their effects. For example, "I allow my physical body to clear from it toxins that have been buried deep within it, and I no longer question the reason for the clearing now." He said etheric body work would further facilitate what he had done.

When I asked about the Rochlitz exercises, Vywamus replied they were excellent, but the issue was neither my immune system nor my physical strength. He said the issue was my attitude. He noted I often approached what I did with a mental intensity which tended to be critical and unloving of myself. He said when working with the immune system, one needed to work with it with love, not intensity, not by saying, "We're going to build you up so that when you're attacked we can make sure you can withstand it." He encouraged me to have compassion for myself and my body, including its role in the clearing process. He added that while my body had been very supportive of me during this lifetime, my attitude during my illness tended to be, "How dare you have any issues to show me . . . deal with it yourself."

Vywamus felt my mental intensity tended to disrupt the healing process. He said I often wanted to heal myself quickly but then did not experience the feelings and bodily sensations which were being reflected back to me. As a result of trying to speed up my healing and not connecting to my body, I did not learn what was to be learned and had to repeat the process over and over and over and over and over and over.

As an alternative, he suggested the next time my body reacted to something, I thank it for the clearing and encourage it to continue if needed. Then I should focus on my internal environment. What was I thinking when I got the reaction? Where had I been? Had I been in my mind? Or had I been in my body? Was I avoiding something? Was that why I was getting the reaction? If I started paying attention to what was going on inside me when I had a reaction, that would give me an idea of what it was I was trying to learn that I did not quite get yet.

By focusing within when I had a reaction, I would learn about thoughts or feelings I was avoiding which needed attention. Vywamus said my soul had created an extraordinary opportunity where I could take time to deal with what was going on inside, but I preferred to approach my illness from a surface viewpoint. He recommended that rather than trying to control my external environment, which I was quite completely focused on, I should respond directly to internal cues as they presented themselves.

When I asked Vywamus about my work, he said the question was premature. First, I had major choices to make about how I was going to connect with myself. The choices I made would determine the direction my work would take. What I had to do was to embrace who and what I was. The three most important areas included seeing my physical body as part of myself, recognizing that when I focused on mental activity I failed to give myself much love and compassion, and listening to what was going on inside of me. He again admonished me to be aware of my feelings and to respond to those internal cues rather than trying to control my external environment. The whole process of my illness had been sensitizing me to this internal focus, but I had to be willing to go through it. At that point time was up.

The hour passed swiftly but affected me for weeks. As soon as I put down the phone, Patricia wanted to know about the session. I sensed it had been helpful but felt too depressed to speak. I shook my head. No, I did not want to talk about it. I then retreated to my room. Vywamus had made a direct assault on defenses I had not even known existed. Although my mind questioned his statements, the feelings of guilt and shame they evoked suggested their accuracy. I spent the next three days in my room pondering how I could live with this dark side of myself which Vywamus had exposed.

Patricia spoke with Vywamus shortly thereafter. She had no way of knowing the content of my session, but it was clear the conversation had devastated me. As she approached her session, Patricia became increasingly apprehensive about what would happen.

She had made a detailed list of questions and began with one about her health. Vywamus responded by saying, "Just don't quite want to be here, eh? . . . Yes, I think that is the problem here." He said there was a tendency to believe that if she really allowed herself to be fully here and fully participate in life on Earth that somehow she would become trapped, she would not be appreciated, and that she would lose her light. She believed she would lose her sensitivity and her ability to connect to spirit and that she would become suffocated in Earth living. Because of these beliefs every time her soul pushed to increase the light in her body she resisted the flow into life. At the same time she eliminated different potentials and opportunities because of her beliefs which said she could not do this or that because it would penetrate her light and her light would not be able to protect itself.

Patricia had never thought of herself as having light and did not understand what Vywamus was saying. Only briefly in her late twenties had she tried meditation, but shortly thereafter her life fell apart. She then spent years trying to regroup. During that time she developed environmental illness. Although she had always been unconsciously and inexplicably drawn toward the mystical, the little dabbling she did had such intense repercussions that she had chosen to stay far away from it. She felt overwhelmed by what Vywamus was saying to her now and struggled to pay attention.

Expecting Vywamus to talk about her childhood, Patricia asked when this belief began. Instead Vywamus told her that where she came from originally, her energy structure was very delicate and refined. When she first approached Earth, it was of a much different vibration than now; and things seemed fine. Repeated experiences with the heavy energy and the denial present on the Earth led to Patricia's having feelings of being contaminated, but by then she could not leave. She began to regret her decision to come to Earth and chose to hold back as much of her light as possible and only contaminate (as she saw it) a little piece of her light.

Vywamus said the basis of her illness was a struggle between the part of her self which was coming from a very high level, seeking to express itself, and the other part, more connected with her soul and Earth living, insisting it was not going to contaminate itself. This battle intensified each time she sought to do something new and different, each time she sought to bring forth more of who she was. He said because she held that belief she had many experiences in many lifetimes which validated it.

Vywamus talked to her about a fear she had of being stuck and told her she had manifested that fear in a variety of ways in different lifetimes, including becoming caught in a sticky, tarlike resin in a jungle. As a result she had developed a great fear of anything which had an energy that she perceived as being sticky, including people who were very physical or very emotional. Instead she gravitated toward relationships where there was a mental clarity. He said she had literally created an allergic reaction to life here on Earth, because Earth living had the potential of getting her stuck. At the same time she was seeking to understand and go beyond these experiences and bring forth who she really was on this plane. He added that, try as she might, she would not be able to avoid this sticky energy, because it is everywhere; and she needed to learn to interact with it. He suggested she did not have to get stuck in it, and that it did not contaminate her if she did not believe so.

Vywamus told Patricia that when she had an allergic reaction, she should observe herself and what was going on around her. Because she had the commonly held belief that people are only allergic to physical things, when she had a reaction she always looked for the physical thing that was the cause. She should give herself permission to see that perhaps she had allergic reactions not so much to physical flows as to emotional flows. She also should pay attention to when the sensitivities or allergies stepped up and allow herself to recognize that they were part of a protective mechanism which she had set up. Now, however, she experienced them as incapacitating, because they locked her in a box which was too small for her. He predicted that if she would deal with the emotional stuff, her allergies would fall away.

He said that when he looked at her physical structure, her body was simply trying to do what she wanted it to. Since she had a very difficult time on an energetic and emotional level saying no, her body was attempting to set her boundaries for her. It created situations in which it said, "No," and she could not move.

He went on to say that 65 to 70 percent of Patricia's illness at that point was continuing out of a codependent need she had to support me. She was so sensitive to other people's energetic flows and responses that if they were not able to receive her love or support on an emotional or a physical level, she would support them by creating the same response inside herself which the other person had inside themselves in order to say, "See you are not alone, I am here."

He explained that although she viewed this as supporting those she interacted with, she was actually taking away from them an opportunity to see things differently. By not sharing her interpretation, not sharing what she saw which was different from others, she could become karmically connected, not by something she did or said, but by something she did not do or say. Vywamus felt this had happened with Patricia and me in the past, and that we were currently repeating an entire relationship. He said this wasn't even new. We had done it before, and it was time to change. Patricia needed to start being herself and stop being my reflection.

Patricia found these comments most confusing. She asked, since she had environmental illness before I did, wasn't this backwards? Vywamus insisted the roles were not reversed. He added that this codependent component altered her ability to heal herself. She could have what she would consider a miraculous recovery if she allowed herself to change the way she related to me and others. She needed to give herself permission to do what she wanted to do and feel what she wanted to feel, rather than being a major support mechanism for those she cared about.

Vywamus repeated that the roles were not reversed. The relationship had brought the opportunity for deep emotional clearing for both of us, but that I simply did not want to deal with much of the physical and emotional parts of who I was. He asked Patricia to look at what she thought my response would be if she woke up one day totally well, totally free of the illness. He suggested I would probably be very angry.

Vywamus suggested Patricia give herself permission to feel energetically when she became aware of the sticky energy. Before she went into "overwhelm," she should let herself quiet down inside and feel how she was interacting on an energetic level. He gave her a meditation to do each morning which would help her set her energetic boundaries.

He reminded her that this was all a choice. She did not have to become involved with another person's energy if she did not want to. She also did not have to process their energy for them just because they were too frightened to process it themselves. Vywamus said Patricia compulsively did this not only with those she loved but also with complete strangers. He advised that Patricia ask Adriana to help her begin to identify the energy by having Adriana send energy to her to see if she could feel it.

By then Patricia felt she was not understanding at all what Vywamus was saying. She figured by later listening to the tape Pat was making of the session, she would comprehend what had been said.

Going back to her, now silly-seeming, list of questions, Patricia skipped over several and asked why she was losing or breaking everything she owned—her glasses and clothing, for starters. Vywamus replied she was trying to magnify the pattern of pushing everything which had to do with the Earth away from her so she could see the pattern clearly. It was a playing out of the part that really did want to be here, really did want clothes, a car, and so on, and the part that did not want to be here. They were playing against one another and asking her to decide. Vywamus said Patricia had not really made her decision about whether or not she wanted to be here. He added it did not matter which choice she made as long as she stood behind the choice 100 percent. Patricia felt slapped in the face by this statement. No one had ever said anything like that to her before.

Vywamus warned her of the need to deal with all of these issues of her internal pollution before we moved to another house, because if *she* did not, if *we* did not, wherever we went we would simply manifest very rapidly that which we were seeking to run from. He asked her to consider that this was what had happened in the house where we were living. He suggested she start thinking about the type of life she wanted to live, to make believe she had none of the problems she now had, and to really allow herself to know what she wanted. He suggested there was a level of fear about doing what she really wanted to do and that much of her illness, her confusion, and her frustration with the environment were ways of taking her attention away from what she really needed to look at.

Vywamus noted that while Patricia's energy structure appeared delicate, she was really very strong. He said she and I were wonderful creators. We had created such a convoluted flow that we would kill ourselves before we looked at what really needed to be looked at, but it was time to start looking at how we would make our lives different if environmental illness were not a problem and then start actively doing that. Then we might find that environmental illness no longer was a problem. With this statement the reading ended.

Patricia was stunned by this conversation. She could not remember most of what Vywamus said but cried for days after her session. She could not stop thinking about the idea that she did not want to exist on the Earth. Patricia was deeply troubled by it but also recognized its accuracy. She acknowledged she felt it did not matter whether she lived or not and admitted to herself how much she hated her job, her illness, and her powerlessness. Her life revolved around environmental illness. She began to see the investment she had in maintaining it and that she had no idea what she would do if she were not ill. Patricia was too ashamed to tell me Vywamus' statement that she was staying sick to support me.

When I finally emerged from my room, I was ready to work with Vywamus' recommendations. I allowed myself to focus more on my body and inner sensations. Becoming aware of feelings of deep sadness and self-hatred, I wondered where they came from. Memories surfaced of my mother's depression and my father's simmering rage, which he held in check except for rare explosive outbursts.

A few days later, Patricia and Adriana tried the exercise suggested by Vywamus. Adriana chose to send her heart energy. Patricia expected to have a pleasant experience but noticed only a subtle sensation around her head which she did not have words to describe. She was astonished a few hours later when a red rash, roughly in the shape of a heart, appeared on her chest. For days her sensitivities to chemicals and foods worsened. Muscle testing indicated Patricia's Candida had flared up. She took this as a demonstration of how taking on energy from others was one way she made herself sick.

As we attended more to our bodies, we noticed several changes. The more we focused on them, the more they communicated with us through various symptoms. The first ones were itchy, red rashes. Patricia's started on her feet and over several months progressed segmentally up her legs, trunk, and arms, sparing her face. Mine began on my legs and buttocks. Simultaneously, we had increased energy and decreased sensitivity to chemicals. For the first time in two years, we were able to spend three hours shopping in malls with minimal difficulty.

This improvement encouraged us to continue exploring the inner dimensions of environmental illness, but often we felt lost as to what we were doing. The trips to the Red House were particularly difficult. We went there once or twice a week to do our laundry and to pack. Our functioning was severely limited if we stayed longer than twenty-four hours. We assumed our aching muscles and clouded thinking were caused by the mold. Our movements were slowed to the point it felt like we were moving through sludge. As we slowed down, I let myself experience the various sensations and emotions that arose, rather than denying them or avoiding them as I had done in the past. Patricia tried, but her joint and muscle aching was so intense that she was not able to be aware of much else. She just wanted the pain to go away.

Our experiences were magnified by having so much to do in the limited time we were able to function at the Red House. We worried about how we would get out of there by the mid-April deadline. Each week the first priority was doing our laundry, consisting of towels and any clothes we could still wear. We no longer had sheets to wash, because ours had been ruined by chemicals, and we slept without any.

Goaded by patients' repeated questions about why Patricia always wore the same jumper, we continued trying to salvage her ozone-damaged clothing. When multiple and varied forms of washing failed, we pursued a friend's suggestion to boil them in salt water. We used the electric burners from our macrobiotic diet days together with two large lobster pots bought specifically for the task. After clearing a foot of snow off the slate patio, we put the burners on it, filled the pots with salted boiling water, and added the clothes. We then took turns in the frigid February air stirring pots of boiling clothes. I asked myself how I had gotten into such a bizarre situation where it was increasingly difficult to accomplish routine tasks like doing laundry and having clothes to wear. After a couple weeks we had to admit boiling was another failure. It discolored and destroyed all but one of the pieces of clothing we tried it on.

In spare moments we packed. Because we suspected many of our possessions had been contaminated by mold, we took special precautions. Everything went into plastic trash bags before going into cardboard boxes. We then drove the boxes to a storage locker in Waltham, a suburb west of Boston. We later learned of others with environmental illness who were familiar with the scenario of mold, plastic bags, and storage lockers.

After updating our list of requirements for a safe house, we briefly tried house hunting again. Our healing had progressed to a point that the list could be less restrictive than in 1990. Since mold had so profoundly disrupted our lives, avoiding it was now a top priority. After the first two rentals we looked at had damp, moldy basements, we decided to postpone our search. We chose to put whatever we wanted to keep in storage and then use the apartment as a base for our housing search after we were out of Great Barrington.

As we went about our daily activities, we continued to become aware of the ways our handling energetic exchanges with others caused us problems. Patricia came home from work one Friday complaining of back pain. Muscle testing indicated she had taken on the pain from a coworker who was having back problems. Patricia felt much better after she used her breath to release the pain as Adriana had showed her. The next day when I returned home from doing psychiatric consultations, Patricia had another intense reaction. Shortly after I walked in the door, she became extremely agitated and then complained of nausea, dizziness, and weakness. Muscle testing showed she was reacting to energies I was still carrying from the people I had evaluated. After I cleared my aura, I felt lighter and more energetic and Patricia's reaction dissipated.

# CHAPTER TEN

# Going Deeper

On February eighth, I had a follow-up session with Vywamus through Pat Balzer over the phone. I expected positive feedback for the gains I had made through my commitment to forging a new relationship with my body and feelings. He quickly set me straight.

Vywamus agreed I had made an effort to become more aware of these parts, but added that awareness was not enough. I had to put into action the information he had given me in January. That was how I was going to make changes so that this new relationship was no longer an idea but a reality. He estimated I was now aware of 5 percent of what was going on inside me.

He asked what I had done since we last talked to simply be with my body. After I told him, he said I still needed to do more. I had only touched the surface of it and my mind wanted to say I was done, that it was time to move on to something else. Vywamus said that was my mind speaking—I needed to allow myself energetically to move more into my body.

Vywamus said I had not yet developed the feeling I needed to really connect with the inner parts of myself. How would I get the feeling? By wanting it. I had not yet quite seen the need to be in my body. He added I had a deep-seated attitude of questioning whether it was worth my while to feel the inner parts of myself. He suggested I needed to become aware of the amount of thoughts I was thinking. He recommended I allow myself to clearly watch the perception inside of self. I needed to allow myself to start feeling things rather than just thinking things. And I needed to allow myself to get into my body. How? By taking up a sport or getting body work or anything else that would get me into my body and then processing what came up when I allowed myself to feel what it was like to be in a body.

He spoke of the importance of getting into a feeling mode to experience my feelings. Because of a reluctance to do so, my mind kept wanting to go further, even though I had not yet done what was needed in order to make the full step. My mind was not able to explore my feelings. I could only do so by feeling them. He suggested reading *Right Use of Will* by Ceanne DeRohan to start me on what I had to do; it would also keep my mind busy. I was bridging a gap in connecting to the feeling level and it would take some time to bring my involvement there up to the kind of connection I had to mind and spirit. He said I was trying to bridge a gap which had existed for a very long time, and it was not going to happen in a week. He encouraged me to work with each body in its own way and to notice when I slipped back into approaching them through my mind. I had to give myself permission to realize that what I was moving here was not my mind.

When asked about the causes of environmental illness, Vywamus replied that there are many frameworks and he would elaborate on three main ones. First, he said that for many people there simply is a disconnection from the physical. The body is seen as something which is pulling the person back, holding them back. The body is viewed as not being as Divine as spirit and mind. It is something that is "less than." For a second group, there is reluctance to allow a full expression on the physical plane, for fear that if we allow full expression, if we fully connect to physicality, somehow we will be judged, criticized, and then will be rejected. For a third group, as they touch into physicality, they do not really wish to own their choice of being here. They will use physicality and they will use many created illnesses and diseases to disconnect them, to create a smokescreen that will take up all their time and energy rather than really being here. So they spend all their money and time worrying about how they are going to connect with this and how this is not connecting to them. They never do anything;

they never fulfill purpose.

Vywamus noted that the presentation in environmental illness varies widely. He also pointed out that while Patricia and I manifested similar symptoms, we each were working on different issues. He compared this situation to that with the English language. You have a limited number of words in the English language, and you can put them together in many different ways to create the effect you want. Similarly, there is a limited amount of disease you can get, and you can play it out any way you want. We would like to think there is only one disease per one type of framework or one type of mindset, and that is not true.

Trying to get some practical help, I asked about the itchy red rash which covered my legs, arms, trunk, and back. He replied the rash reflected my body's anger and irritation at me for having failed to listen to it for so long. Vywamus predicted the rash was going to get a lot worse before it got better. He said the rash also was a clearing, a releasing of emotions, and a concurrent wanting to crawl out of my skin, a wanting to create something else to get away from the feelings. He added that before I could heal my body, I would have to make friends with it. He asked if I thought my body wanted to be scratched or if my scratching was an attempt to make the irritation and the feelings go away. Vywamus again stressed the importance of allowing feelings in my body to surface and owning any feelings I had toward it.

One way to see what was going on inside was to look at what my body was showing me and then react to it and own my response. He said I had been so blaming my problems on the environment that I did not see I was also blaming my body. He said I held such thoughts as, "I don't like this itching. Why do you have to itch? You're always bugging me. Look at you! You're always constantly irritating me. Why can't you do anything right?" He added that I was unaware of these feelings and needed to allow them to become conscious. Once I owned what I was feeling, things could shift quite rapidly and completely. Until I did so, a shift could not occur.

At the end of the half-hour session, I asked about the different spiritual paths which people follow, how some focus on the light and exclude any consideration of the dark side of things while others emphasize an interplay of light and darkness. Vywamus answered that those focusing on the light *or* the dark were working in a polarized state, eliminating all possible contamination of the other. Eventually, the last step at the end would be to shoot into the other path to accept it fully. At that point there would be a blending of the two. Or you could step in a path where you have one foot in the light and one foot in the dark so that a blending occurred along the way. This path moved through the body which was to be embraced without judgment.

Since I was here in a body and was not leaving it, Vywamus recommended I put one foot in the body. He said once I truly embraced my body unconditionally and without judgment, the body would come into alignment with me and embrace me completely; there would be no separation. I would move beyond body and mind and simply be ONE.

I asked again what I should do. He said I needed to commit to being in my body. Once I did that I would commit to being in the NOW. As I committed to being in the NOW, I would commit to the experiential path. Then it would not matter what I did, what work I did. I would simply do what I wanted to do and from that I would learn about myself. I had not gained that learning experience, because I had not been committed to being in my body and in the NOW; but I would as I sought to go beyond that which had been. I felt far from that experience.

After I hung up the phone, I started judging myself again. I told myself I had been wasting my time trying to relate to my body. I felt discouraged that I had made so little progress. At the same time from somewhere deep inside me arose the desire to truly connect with my body, but I did not know how I would do that. Perhaps in addition to being a major source of discomfort and aggravation the rash was my body's way of communicating with me. When I asked what my body wanted, an inner voice replied, "to be massaged regularly, including self-massage every day." I committed myself to doing that.

As Vywamus brought the inner origins of Patricia's and my illness to our awareness, we at times had alarming exacerbations of our sensitivities. One day when I went to my Watertown Square post office box, I was confronted by a harsh chemical odor which sent my muscles into spasm and brought on nausea. It smelled like someone had poured concentrated cleaning fluid on the floor and then failed to rinse it off. I hurriedly emptied my box and left, but the strong smell was now on my mail. From the pain in my muscles I knew I could not tolerate leaving the letters in my car while I drove to work. Instead, I went home and put the mail in the back room window, between the glass and screen, to air it out.

When I told Patricia about this episode, we were perplexed as to what had happened. Were the cleaning products in the post office that toxic? I had not noticed that smell before. Or had I suddenly become more sensitive to those products, too? The next day I called the post office manager and told him about my reactions. I expressed concern not only about my health but also about the safety of other customers and his employees. He agreed to do what he could to correct the situation. Even with the adjustments he made, the mail still reeked of the cleaner smell and had to be aired before being brought into the apartment.

On February twelfth Patricia had her second session with Vywamus. She told him she had done the meditation he suggested but felt it had not helped her. He replied that the process was going to take time. He described how she had been using her body as a barometer without recognizing she was doing so. There was a disconnect between the conscious mind and the energy she was playing in. She was not observing the energetic flows, and this was creating problems with maintaining her energetic field. Now the body was mirroring this disconnection so she would pay attention.

When she complained that she could not feel the energetic flows, Vywamus launched into a discussion about her programming, her mental body, and its intention to take charge of the other aspects of self. He said she was able to sense these flows, but she judged and questioned what she sensed. Her mental body needed constant verification of what was going on in her energy field. He said when someone has a problem with boundaries, it is because the mental body has to be in charge; and it cannot say no unless it sees good logic in saying no. The mental body does not allow the emotional body or the physical body to come forth and set boundaries unless there is a good logical reason for it.

She had in this and other lifetimes attempted to eliminate input from the other bodies of self and to depend completely on the mental body, but there are certain areas the mental body cannot get a handle on. Therefore the mental body says these things do not matter. This attitude has major effects on the other bodies.

Vywamus told Patricia she did not trust what she could not see clearly through the mental body and had created a fragmented state. In the mental body's opinion, since the other bodies are not valid and cannot do the job appropriately, it will figure out the way to do things right. However, it can't because it's working in an area in which it has no expertise. It has no sense, no ability, no way to measure it, no way to understand it, no way to allow itself to participate in the flow of the emotional body, because it is not in the emotional body. Patricia was going to have to give herself permission to let go of the need to quantify her choice, to allow herself to make the choice without the backup of the logic, then simply begin acting on it.

He said that in the process of developing environmental illness she had a major fragmentation inside which said the problem existed, so it would not automatically go away. As she hung onto that belief—as she committed to it—and as she tried on the other hand to shift it, it was going to be a process where she eventually came to the conclusion that no one was causing her problems except herself, and her perceptions of how it was caused would become the reality of it. Since that would take a while, she would see a gradual lessening and as she got to certain points there would be integrations. Then she would see an increase in the problems, but only because the thought form would be frightened to fully acknowledge that this did not have anything to do with anyone attacking her.

He elaborated by saying that when Divinity believes it is whole, it is completely connected to itself and no attack-defense is set up. There is no need for an attack-defense system because it is not fighting against itself. When Divinity splits up, it tries to prove that one piece is bigger or better or one piece is lesser or worse than the other; then you have to set up a whole attack-defense system. That was what had happened in her energetic field and that had been translated into her physical body and its environment. So it is in recognizing that when you are truly connected to yourself, there is no need to fend off or to create a reaction to yourself. In full connection there is a complete honoring of self, regardless of what self chooses to be or take on or do at that moment. It gets very interesting in that process, and that was the process Patricia was attempting to move through.

Vywamus said her situation involved long-standing fragmentation, and there had been a long-standing attempt to support the belief that her self was not whole, that the Earth was attacking her, that she was fragmenting here, she was away from their center. It was going to take a great deal of conscious alignment with herself to shift this. One way for her to begin to shift it was to give herself permission to be very careful with what she was thinking. She should monitor her thoughts carefully and notice when she attacked herself.

By "attacking herself," Vywamus said he meant *doubting* herself. He explained that doubt was an attack on self. When you doubt yourself, you take a piece of self, put it on a pedestal, and ask yourself if this piece is valid. By simply thinking, "Is this piece valid?" you are already thinking it is not. Each time you doubt yourself, it is a disconnect, an invalidation, and a support of this attack-defense mechanism, or "gapping," which is taking place inside of self.

Vywamus pointed out to Patricia that doubt, criticism, and self-judgment were very conscious. Because they were so conscious, she thought of them as a natural part of her essence. Therefore, she did not pay attention to them. He said there was a conscious choice to deny the conscious choice here. Eventually, the struggle had to play itself out in her physical body, so that she could see it clearly. He added that if someone were to cut up a being from another planet or a little child, and look at it, examine it, and invalidate it the way she had done to herself, she would be outraged.

Patricia then told Vywamus of the bloodless image of the baby chopped into pieces which she had seen during her MariEL treatment. Vywamus responded that was what she did to herself. He added that she was so disconnected from what she was doing to herself and she did it with such a lack of compassion that she saw no blood. She saw no pain. She felt no pain. That came from eons of doing it. That was why it was layered into her physical body the way it was. Vywamus added that she was not the only one to do this; everyone does it. In fact, most people are in her situation. They have gone completely numb to what it feels like to be hurt. In her recovery process, there was a part of her which was going numb to it and the other part was waking up to it and seeking to correct that which had been done.

Vywamus said that you work backward through the process when you went to sleep. The last thing you numbed out to was how it felt and that's the first thing you wake up to. Part of the process of moving into that recognition is moving into the stage in which you tend to project the attack on self out onto everyone else and feel completely victimized by those people in your life who have "done it to you," have mirrored to you what you have done to yourself.

As you sit in that pain, you eventually get to the point where you recognize it is not going to change anything; and you decide you no longer need the pain to see what you are feeling. You begin to recognize that the reason the pain is there is because you chose the feeling and you chose the action. You begin to see how you have done it to yourself, and you draw that fragment which you have placed outside yourself back in where you begin to resolve it within yourself. At that point, you recognize what you have done and that it was a choice to do it. Then you choose *not* to do it. The whole issue—be it related to parents, friends, partners, abuse, abandonment, whatever—is completely transmuted instantaneously, and in your memory there is no more pain. There is simply an experience from which you learned.

Vywamus went on to say pain is only present when there is a gap, when there has been a separation between you and wholeness. Pain is simply joy that has been fragmented. When you bring yourself back together, the pain transmutes into joy. And you begin to see— "Look what have I done!"—and you become aware of the choices. Eventually, you will no longer see it as a choice that you have to fight against. You simply choose not to treat yourself that way.

Vywamus repeated that this process would take a while and would require a conscious commitment to go beyond the point where one is at and not simply take a fix-it attitude so that you can get to the next point. He emphasized that the only way Patricia was going to heal this was to be absolutely in the NOW, because in the NOW there is no way to deny the pain. The pain, be it physical or emotional, was the key to what she was doing, how she was fragmenting herself. If there is pain, you know you are fragmenting, but you cannot experience that unless you are in the absolute NOW.

Vywamus predicted it was going to take practice; Patricia was not going to get it right away. It was going to take practice, then she would forget, then she would remember, then she would practice again, and each time, she was going to practice a little more. Simply sitting down once a day and doing a meditation was not going to do it. Patricia needed to do this process actively in her everyday life.

When Patricia asked about her rash, Vywamus answered it was an irritation about her own nurturing process. There was a part of her that was *so* intent on nurturing herself *so* perfectly. The intention and her concept of perfection came from a very judgmental state. There was recognition of this on some level and great rage and disgust at self for what she was doing to herself. Because the mind exerted too much control to let her rage come out any other way, it came right out through the skin. Vywamus added there was still the belief of "look at what the body is doing to me now."

Vywamus advised that Patricia give herself permission to become very sensitive to her feelings, to try to feel them, and to act on them without having to mentally justify it to herself. He said MariEL could help her release the patterned response of her mental logic and free up the compulsive need to assess everything.

Once again Patricia felt totally at a loss, unable to understand much of anything Vywamus had said to her. She wondered why she had ever agreed to have a second reading with him. Unable to think clearly, she returned to her list of questions.

She described a vivid dream she had in 1990, in which the two of us were in Africa doing healing work. We were surrounded by many children. The dream had haunted Patricia, leaving her with the distinct feeling that it had an important symbolic meaning which she had yet to understand. She asked Vywamus for his input.

He replied that before Patricia began working as a healer, she needed to heal her own womb—her own feminine; to go deep within and nurture herself, and in doing so she would open up to her own healing abilities. He cautioned she must allow herself to be herself, because her healing abilities were not going to frame in through the mind, not even going to come anywhere near the mind. If she tried logically to detect and measure them and prove they were present, she would literally suffocate them.

Vywamus said Africa represented the Black Continent, the unlimited potentiality, the rawness of Mother Earth. That was where much of Patricia's denial lay and where much of her power lay. He said she needed to go back home to find her power. Vywamus said Patricia needed to come back home to herself, to love herself, to nurture all of herself, not just little bits and pieces of herself. She needed to be who she was completely. Vywamus predicted that if she allowed that to take place, everything would flow in quite easily. Her healing process would be quite amazing, and there would not have to be a lot of struggle. The way to get to that point was being in the NOW, and he encouraged Patricia to practice being in the NOW. With that advice the session ended.

Patricia hung up the phone feeling even more dumbfounded

than after her first reading. What had he said? How could she ever make sense of all that? How was she going to get well? He said she was a healer! Was she?

The following evening I spoke with Vywamus for another half hour. He said he had broken my second reading with him into two sessions, because he knew I would need to think about what we had discussed and would have questions. He was right. My mind filled with questions as I contemplated moving beyond it into my body and my feelings.

He told me in several different ways that I needed to slow down and let go of my judging process. He added that it was going to take time to go beyond the mental understanding of what he was saying and to truly layer the understanding into my full perspective so I would not forget again. He said I wanted to bypass the body and move on to the next thing and get bigger and better. He further described my mental intensity and my need to know more as having an addictive quality and that these behaviors were ways to avoid dealing with what was underneath. He said they came from an inability to connect with the rest of self.

Vywamus indicated that I could learn what I needed to know in a very short time, that it did not need to be dragged on for weeks or months at a time. He said I tended to interpret mental intensity as learning, but much of what is learned that way is easily forgotten— as in an intense course one would study and take an exam for. With true experiential learning, the learning comes quickly and is not forgotten—like riding a bicycle or learning to walk. Once you get it, you do not forget it.

He talked about the importance of allowing myself to feel, because this was how I would get in touch with my will. Many people *think* their feelings rather than *feel* their feelings, because they have a great deal of judgment on specific feelings. By thinking their feelings they can avoid certain flows of energy which don't fit into their concepts of right and wrong. When people think their feelings, there is the presence of guilt and blame.

In response to my question about the effectiveness of various schools of psychology in working with feelings, Vywamus said those disciplines are created to support what one believes. Very few disciplines really support feeling feelings. In fact, very few disciplines support really looking at and acknowledging what is present, and truly honoring and loving it without trying to making something right. Many disciplines, whether psychological or spiritual, actually have a layer of judgment over them regarding physicality versus spirituality, regarding emotionality versus mentality. He pointed out that although these disciplines have been practiced by many dedicated people, not many people had met ascension in that manner. And, he said, that is why, for all the beautiful disciplines that have been on the Earth for quite some time, the Earth still is layered in a great web of denial and deceit. He added that many times the traditions or disciplines are very appropriate for where you are at the moment. When you are really enmeshed in your patterned responses, these disciplines can give you a little bit of detachment to allow for a greater perspective, which is needed. Once you get that perspective, you need to move on to the next step.

I then asked how Vywamus recommended working with feelings. He answered that feelings are fragmented emotions. When you are looking backward into the wholeness, that is, once you are fragmented, you have to start at the fragment and work your way back to bring it into the wholeness. The first step is feeling and acknowledging, unconditionally allowing the feelings to be there, and allowing self to flow in and out of them, to discover there is nothing to be frightened of. As you release your judgment around this or that feeling, then there is a natural coming together. Once the old charges and judgments have been moved away, you can utilize bridging techniques to take the fragmented feeling state and put it into the whole emotion. He said within the Divine Will there are only five basic emotions. He named them as unconditional love, courage, flow, joy, and compassion. For every feeling there is a polarization. When you put the polarized feelings together, they create part of the wholeness.

When I asked about muscle testing, Vywamus replied it could

be very helpful to connect into points of consciousness which are buried below the mind, to get out of the mind chatter. It works for a while for different parts of the body with which communication is blocked. As soon as communication is opened up, muscle testing is not needed any more; it will be possible to clearly hear what is going on.

He cautioned that many times people use muscle testing when they have a real sense of their own feeling and they do not like the feeling, or they are judging the feeling of not knowing if something is right or wrong. Then when they look to muscle testing for validation, they may get very contradictory flows. He suggested asking the body if it wants muscle testing, regardless of whether or not you think it would be helpful. Otherwise you are still approaching the body as being separated from yourself. Your perception is what is coming through in the muscle testing. Sometimes when there are major judgments layered over the perceptions, these can affect how the tester sees the situation. One needs to be aware of this limitation.

Vywamus thought muscle testing was an excellent way to begin the communication process. It can help get into specific areas you are not yet able to reach intuitively, but it is only a step in the process. But before you can have an intuitive connection, you have to be willing, within the belief structure, to touch the area unconditionally. Intuition is really the spiritual-emotional communication flow. To develop your intuition you want to become very aware of the emotional body. Your intuition is one way Spirit can speak to you without getting fragmented. And the body can be involved with intuition as you allow yourself to sink deeper into it.

Vywamus reminded me that I was always moving exactly as I needed to move, experiencing exactly what I needed to experience, and exactly at the point in the process where I needed to be. If I could simply accept that, then there would be no struggle of whether I was ahead or behind, how well I was doing or when would I get there. There would be an acceptance of the process. If I could surrender to the process and accept that I was exactly where

I needed to be, there would be no need to fight it, no need to defend myself against it, no need to quantify it, to judge it and compare it to my expectations. He said I was getting to that point and we would move as rapidly as we could and no faster.

With that comment my second reading ended. Like Patricia, at the time, I understood little of what was said. I transcribed the tape of my first Vywamus reading and shared it with her. We planned to listen to the other tapes but got caught up in the process of moving and then forgot about them.

On March twenty-first we picked up a fourteen-foot rental truck in Pittsfield to move the first large load of our belongings into storage. It turned out to be another odd encounter reminiscent of "The Twilight Zone." I started the truck and within a few hundred feet of the rental office was overcome by nausea and muscle spasms. Aware of a chemical odor, I drove back to Great Barrington in a disoriented state with Patricia following in the car. She had no idea of the problems I was having and was surprised to see me stagger out of the truck when we reached the house. She was even more surprised to find a paint brush covered with hardened shellac behind the driver's seat! For hours we tried airing the truck out but to no avail. Finally, we turned it in to a local drop-off center the next day. Now we had one less weekend to move. On top of that my winter coat smelled of shellac and provoked symptoms to the point I could not wear it. I improvised by bundling up in layers and hoped spring would arrive soon.

The next Friday we tried renting another truck. I made it clear to the manager we could not tolerate strong odors and chemicals and told him we had to return the previous truck because of the shellac brush left in it. He assured me this one would be fine. When I opened the door, however, I smelled ammonia and other cleaners. I refused to take it. The rental people had no comprehension of the impact of the chemicals they used. No other large truck was available. With two weekends left before the mid-April deadline, we had lost another moving opportunity.

In light of the problems we were having with rental trucks, we questioned whether we would ever escape the Red House. To get a fresh perspective on moving and her health, Patricia had a channeled reading with Helios. Adriana had suggested we might find him easier to speak with than Vywamus. Helios describes himself as the soul aspect of our physical sun, who focuses on opening our hearts into a soul connection, integrating the physical body with the soul aspect of ourselves. Sheila Simon, another resident of the Greenwood House, was the channel.

When Patricia asked about her chronic Candida problem, Helios talked about gaps between the four bodies—physical, mental, emotional, and spiritual—and how they caused health problems like Candida. He said wherever there is an energetic gap, something will come in and fill the space. A lot of her gaps manifested in her belly and these spaces were filled with Candida. He said this had been a problem for her for a long time, but it was starting to get better. It would resolve as she closed the gaps, particularly those between her mental and emotional bodies.

Helios emphasized how important it was for as many people as possible to start releasing the gapping mechanisms very rapidly. The energy referred to in the 11:11 was coming in on increasingly more intense waves. Helios predicted that when the bigger waves came in, anyone still having large gaps would feel like they were being thrown around inside. It would be difficult for them to maintain a place of stability inside themselves. They might develop dizziness, nausea, and other symptoms. Those who released the gaps inside themselves would develop a strong internal base of energy to work from. Then, when the accelerating energy came in, the effect would be soothing, because they would be familiar with it. Rather than being confused or disorganized by the energy, they would be able to embrace it and ground it.

Patricia was especially concerned about the intense itching we were having. As Vywamus predicted, the itching had gotten worse. It interrupted our sleep and interfered with nearly anything else we tried to do. Similar to Vywamus' analysis, Helios said that, on one level, the itching was a clearing of built-up toxicity; on another level, it was a release of anger. He felt we would have it for at least six more months while we closed gaps between our mental and physical bodies. As we released toxic subconscious patterns and got them to move, the physical body would be stimulated to do something with them. Since the skin is the largest breathing organ of the body, it was the easiest way to release the toxicity. Helios strongly recommended we support the physical body in this releasing process rather than trying to suppress the itching.

Patricia next asked about attending a training in MariEL healing scheduled for the following week. She wanted to go but, because of our move, thought waiting for a later one might be better. Helios encouraged her to study MariEL as soon as possible. She would learn how to put an energy grid on her body which would facilitate the clearing process and would stabilize her energetically. Hence her rash and itching would move out more quickly. Knowing MariEL would make it easier to manage the energy changes that would be coming in the months ahead. Helios recommended I take the training too. He said it was important for each of us to develop our own internal support mechanism.

Patricia queried Helios about why we felt so sick in the Red House. He replied that the house had given us the opportunity to see external reflections of ways we internally fragmented ourselves. He said mold overgrowth and sensitivity to it represented unresolved emotional issues and that when we started to "gap" on a mental or emotional level, the house "gapped" on a physical level through mold. Inside us the gapping manifested as Candida. He explained that now when we spent extended periods of time in the house, we again became hooked into the gapping process and became fragmented rather than looking at our experiences from a place of non-judgment.

He predicted that over the next year our physical, mental, emotional, and spiritual bodies would come together so that gapping would no longer occur. Then we would be able to return to the Red House and not be bothered at all. For the present, it was essential we disconnect from the physical structure of the house and let go of the fragmentation it reflected, *before* studying MariEL.

Helios' comments fired up Patricia. When she told me about them, I recoiled and asked how we could move that soon. We had planned to do it over the next two weekends. She replied that Helios said I would question his recommendations and suggested I listen to the session on tape. As I did so, I felt energy shifts in my body reflecting the truth in what he said. Yes, getting out of Great Barrington on Sunday, five days later, and studying MariEL the following night was right for us. I did not know how we would do it.

# CHAPTER ELEVEN

# Letting Go

Helios' comments set off a flurry of activity. To be moved in five days, we needed help. Early Wednesday I made phone calls to see what assistance was available. John Ingersoll, Inc. could provide men who would disinfect items we wanted to keep and then load them onto the moving van. A company called The Master Garbologist could deliver a dumpster so we could discard anything we were not keeping or giving away. Leaving the house and our moldy possessions would be relatively easy. More difficult would be letting go of the limiting beliefs, thought patterns, and emotions which Helios said were reflected in the fragmentation we had experienced living at the Red House.

Friday was one of two days we had set aside for moving. We awoke early and arrived in Great Barrington by eight-thirty. I dropped Patricia off at the house and went to the local Ryder office where I met the Ingersoll men. Jimmy and Matt followed me in the twenty-foot van. After some difficulty navigating the long, winding driveway, Matt backed the truck up twenty feet from the front steps.

Escape from the nightmare house finally seemed possible. The van was there, and in the driveway was a dumpster from The Master Garbologist. I led the men through the house to give them an overview of what needed to be done. I also told them to let us know about items they wanted, because we were giving many things away.

After I showed the men our nontoxic cleaning supplies, they began washing things with disinfectant on the front lawn, drying them, and loading them on the truck. While they did that, Patricia and I made final decisions about what to give away, what to discard, and what to pack. As I went through my possessions, many items triggered memories of a past which now seemed foreign and far away. Environmental illness was the demarcation point. Before it, my life was simple; with it, my life had become an unimaginably complex struggle to survive.

At lunchtime Matt and Jimmy started carting away things they wanted. It felt strange to see them load my favorite sofa onto their pickup. I had chosen the sofa for the rich texture of its plush fabric, but we had not sat on it in over a year. We had tried to protect it from the fleas by putting it in one of the first-floor offices, but now had to assume it was contaminated with mold. They also took the bedroom set that Patricia bought when she moved to Boston. She sensed the furniture represented part of her past which she had to let go, but its departure had a surrealistic quality. She had an image of standing at the edge of a cliff and watching the furniture fall down into a deep, wide canyon. She was giving it away but had nothing to replace it with and no money to buy anything else. Pleased with their windfall, the men returned from lunch with a larger truck to take away more.

Some things had to be thrown away. The organic futon used once on the floor in the family room had developed an unfamiliar smell, which persisted in spite of repeated ozoning and airing. We suspected the smell was from mold or chemicals. Anything made of fabric that could not be washed had to go.

By five o'clock in the afternoon nearly everything we wanted had been cleaned and loaded on the truck. Matt agreed to return on Sunday to help with what remained to be done. After the men left, we worked two hours more before heading back to Watertown.

Saturday was supposed to be a day of rest and recovery. Patricia slept and cooked. I went to the first in a series of four all-day classes given by Andy Cappanigro, a musician turned healer. I decided to take the class after Adriana described him as a western shaman. The teacher, Michael, had said I was on a shamanic journey. Perhaps Andy could help along that path. He specialized in using the breath to release fear and pain through focusing on prana, the energy behind the breath. Andy had found that by freeing the breath, many problems of mind and body could be released.

The first class concentrated on developing greater awareness of the breath when it was restricted by tension and when it was moving freely. We also learned how to use the breath to release stress in ourselves and others. I enjoyed these new ways to facilitate the letting-go process; but when I returned to the apartment, Patricia complained that my energy made her sick. Standing next to me, she felt weak, dizzy, and nauseous. Muscle testing indicated Andy's class had stimulated an intense clearing. In order for Patricia not to be affected she had to stay twenty feet away from me. Not only was this a major problem in the apartment, but we wondered how we would be able to ride in the same car the next day.

We woke early Sunday morning and left Watertown at six o'clock. Fortunately, the clearing process had abated so that we were able to ride together. The windows next to me soon fogged up and stayed that way for the first half of the trip. As we drove 120 miles on the Massachusetts Turnpike to Lee, we recalled the last nineteen months of repeated trips over that road. We had driven it so many times that I now knew the name of every town along the way and the location of every mile marker. We had traveled at all hours of the day and night, in all kinds of weather. It was hard to believe the Great Barrington-part of our ordeal was finally ending.

Going up the driveway for the last time, I wondered why life there had turned out as it had. We had been entranced by the Red House's beautiful mountain setting and moved there with hopes of recovery. But hopes and scenery were not enough. Eventually, we grew to hate it there. All our possessions had either been destroyed by mold or would need extensive treatment before we could use them again. Living there had been a constant drain on our energy and finances.

Upon our arrival at the house, we resumed packing and cleaning. Matt came at noon and brought three friends to gather more booty, including a rocking chair, tables, and an air conditioner. As the men removed them, I reminisced on the use they had given me in the past. Now it was time to let them go.

When Matt left at five o'clock, the heavy lifting was done, but hours of work remained. Throughout the evening we packed boxes and threw things away. By midnight an end was in sight. The remaining letters and mementos were too sacred to throw away. We decided to burn them. Even tolerating a fire was indicative of the progress we had made. Previously, the smoke would have brought on multiple symptoms. After building a fire in the fireplace, we watched the memorabilia go up in smoke and offered thanks for the experiences they represented. We also thanked the Red House for its gifts to us. It had not given us the hoped-for recovery but had pushed us to our limits and beyond, forcing us into realms of healing we otherwise might never have explored.

By three o'clock we were packed and ready to go. I went first in my car. Patricia followed in the truck. Driving through the pitch-black night, I tried to keep sight of her in my rearview mirror and thought of everything we had been through. We had supported each other through the most difficult of times. Yet, ultimately, we each were responsible for our own healing. We each had to choose for ourselves whether or not we wanted to be well.

I stopped in a rest area at mile twenty-nine on the turnpike to check on Patricia and the truck. To my surprise she was not right behind me. I waited as calmly as I could for a few minutes and then began to panic. Where was she? Various images raced through my mind. Normally she would have stopped when I did. Had she been in an accident? Was she hurt? How ironic. We had escaped Great Barrington, and now she had disappeared. I had no way to contact her to learn what had happened.

After meditating for twenty minutes, I was inspired to call our answering machine in Watertown. To my relief, there was a message from Patricia wanting to know what had happened to me. She was parked next to the toll booth in Lee and would not move until she heard from me. My only option was to drive eleven miles east to the next exit, turn around, and then drive thirty miles west to where she was waiting. This early morning driving in circles on the turnpike seemed a fitting conclusion to nineteen months of convoluted chaos in western Massachusetts.

By the time I reached Lee it was five o'clock. What a relief to see Patricia asleep in the truck. After I roused her by tapping on the window, we discussed what to do. We were both exhausted but had to keep going. We had a nine o'clock appointment with movers in Waltham. As we drove east, I made sure to keep her in view. Driving as fast as the fully loaded truck allowed, we arrived in Waltham just before the movers. It took them three hours to unload the truck into storage. Then we returned the truck, drove back to the apartment, and collapsed. We had four hours to rest before the MariEL class that evening.

Helios had said, learning MariEL would speed our healing, and he was correct. The course was given at a MariEL practitioner's home in Acton. Students included a dozen women ranging in age from their twenties to their sixties, Patricia, and myself. None of the others were chemically sensitive. In fact, several reeked of perfume, but the odors did not bother us. Strongly scented items in the house also had no ill effects. Somehow it seemed all the MariEL energy in the house lessened our sensitivity to smells.

Our teacher was Ethel Lombardi, originator of the MariEL healing techniques. She was a light-hearted and vivacious Irish grandmother, who radiated love and enthusiasm. Following a near-death experience at age forty-three, she was miraculously cured of heart disease. She then pursued spiritual studies and in 1976 became a master of Reiki, a form of healing which works with universal life energy. In the early 1980s, she developed MariEL as a fast and powerful form of energetic healing.

The class met over five consecutive evenings. An important focus throughout was learning to give a MariEL treatment. In a treatment, the healer tunes into different areas of the client's body where memories of past traumas from this or previous lives are stored, and proceeds energetically to remove them. The person then gives permission for that area to function in health and joy. We each received at least one treatment. During mine I released emotional pain I had not even realized was present.

We also learned to mentally place a series of lines on our bodies corresponding to new energy pathways. Ethel said they were similar to the meridians found in Oriental medicine but in a very different pattern. She added that these pathways would allow us to flow with and ground the energy that was coming to the Earth.

On the last evening, Ethel told us how she came to develop MariEL healing. She added that the transfer of this energy is assisted by Mother Mary and special angels, called the MariEL healing angels. Ethel's story reminded Patricia of her first MariEL session with Adriana. While lying on the treatment table with her eyes closed, Patricia had seen a beautiful blue light. At first she was reluctant to say anything, but by the end of the session she felt able to mention the light. Adriana replied, matter of factly, that that was Mother Mary. Patricia was stunned by the notion that Mary would help with her healing. Experiences in her catechism classes had left Patricia with unpleasant associations to anything church-related. Adriana emphasized she was talking about the spiritual presence of Mary, not about religious dogma.

The completion of the class marked the end of a whirlwind week. We had extracted ourselves from Great Barrington and taken the basic MariEL training. Putting the MariEL energy grid on every day definitely lessened our symptoms and increased our energy. Now we had to settle into the Watertown apartment and decide what to do next. Would we be safe there or would it be better to move again? If so, where?

Our experiences in several areas suggested we best move soon. Laundry was a prime example. We had done it in Great Barrington until the end. Now our washer and dryer were in storage. We tried the apartment building's laundry facilities, but residual detergent smells bothered me, even when we cleaned the washer first. Patricia tried that washer several times. I could not understand why she risked the few pieces of clothing she was able to wear. Although she could smell residual detergent, she wanted to wear the clothing anyway to see if she could tolerate it. After the detergent smell strongly affected me, I insisted we not use those machines.

Patricia's friend Joan let us use her new washer and agreed to use our detergent to keep the washer safe for us. She also offered use of her new dryer, but its chemicals proved too much. As an alternative we resorted to a clothesline strung across the living room. In the past, friends had commented on how neat my apartment was. Now it was in constant disarray with laundry drying in the living room and our possessions strewn throughout.

For direction as to what to do next, I spoke with Helios through Sheila. I asked about the last two years, which I had experienced as a breaking down of my physical body. He replied that although I had focused on changes in my physical body, much release had occurred on other levels, including the mental. He added that whatever was going on in my physical environment, whatever was going on in my emotional body and in my physical body, mirrored back to me what was going on in my mental body.

He said I had to realize that I had been given the opportunity to see externally how different internal structures I had created over an extended period of time did not create wholeness. The house in Great Barrington had shown us all the aspects of self that were an illusion and did not support us. In doing so, it had created a clearing for us. Helios chided me, saying I had stubbornly resisted the process. He added that, for many people, in order to get them to look at areas where they had been in denial for a long time, it had been necessary for their soul to create situations from which they could not escape. In those situations they became deeply intertwined with shadow aspects of themselves. Then the situation magnified the imbalances in such an extreme manner on an external level that it caused an internal breakdown.

Helios indicated that many others were going through a similar process. Ours had manifested as environmental illness. Theirs might take different forms. The common theme was a need to release structures that were created inside of self as a place to hide which, if left untouched, continued to create the destructive thought patterns of the past.

When I asked how people in general would experience these effects, Helios replied that they might say nothing they had done in the past worked anymore. Or they might say they felt like all the different systems that exist, such as the political system, the economic system, and the health-care system, do not work anymore and these individuals do not know what to do about it. Many would feel lost. Helios said that with the work Patricia and I had been doing with Adriana and other healers, as well as with Vywamus and MariEL, we were starting to come out the other side of this process.

I then questioned Helios about what would help others during this period of massive change. He answered first that you cannot take away their pain—they need to learn whatever they need to learn. All you can do is show them either verbally or through healing that whatever they are resisting is what they need to surrender to; as long as they continue fighting this energy, fighting this breakdown inside themselves or in various systems, trying to make life the way it used to be, the more pain they are going to create for themselves.

As the session came to a close, I sought Helios' advice regarding where to live. Would it be beneficial to stay in the Watertown apartment for a while or was it better to move? He recommended we find a place away from the city, especially as a place to be in the summer months. A windy place with constant air movement instead of the urban stagnation would be best. More direct contact with the earth would also aid in the clearing process. He suggested we begin looking in Scituate, Wayland, and Sharon.

Helios ended by saying Patricia and I were doing well. He stressed the importance of continuing to simplify rather than complicate our lives, having a clear focus in whatever we did, and dropping the mental body down inside of self instead of being focused only in the head. When we listened to the tape of the reading, we appreciated its broad perspective on the process we had been going through.

We were slowly getting better. I could now drive without a barrier cloth or cotton gloves. Patricia was feeling more energetic. We would rather take a break from moving, but we also wanted to be out of the city by summer. As a compromise we decided to delay house hunting for a few weeks.

The next Saturday was the final class with Andy Cappanigro. I again wanted to use a barrier cloth to protect myself from the fumes of his new carpet. By using the barrier cloth and sitting near an open window, I had felt reasonably comfortable during our previous meetings. Andy had hitherto allowed me to take these measures but now insisted I do without the barrier cloth. He said using it just reinforced my illness. Although I followed his direction, I felt angry and misunderstood.

At the end of the day, students gave Andy feedback. Many praised him for what they had learned. When my turn came, the fury which had simmered in me all day exploded in a torrent of anger directed at him. Its intensity was surprising, but behind the anger I felt a reservoir of power inside myself. Andy responded by saying that I suppressed my anger and in doing so dampened my energy. He added that feeling my emotions instead of "going passive" to them would be strengthening for me.

I listened to his comments but was so enraged that concentrating was impossible. I left as soon as the class ended. When I told Patricia what had happened, she said she thought I had overreacted. She agreed that it might be time to let go of the barrier cloth, that it did reinforce my illness. The next morning I followed Andy's suggestion of tuning into any anger and irritability inside myself and allowing it to be. As I did so and focused on my breath, I felt both an easing of tension and renewed energy flowing through me. Only months later would I acknowledge Andy's skill as a shaman. He had poked and prodded me in a way that brought my rage to the surface.

The theme of releasing rage appeared again the following Saturday during a one-day workshop on healing that was held at the Greenwood House. We had a discussion about the healing process and then worked with sound and movement to help us get into our bodies and ground our energy. The rest of the day we did bodywork in groups of four or five.

For weeks after the workshop, our itching was unbearable. Patricia would start cooking dinner each evening around six o'clock but we might not eat until hours later. She frequently ended up in a corner, crying and scratching herself, sometimes drawing blood. Helios reminded us the itching was a way of releasing rage and would continue until we learned to express it in other ways, because the body was no longer willing to hold it. He also told us that as we continued to heal, our energy bodies were expanding rapidly, often creating a lot of heat. These changes contributed to a rapid clearing through the skin, producing the rash and itching. Helios suggested things to help cool the body down like eating cooling foods, swimming in Walden Pond, taking cold showers, or having a cold soak in the bathtub. Several times Patricia ended up putting ice cubes in the tub to calm her skin down.

Helios also recommended that Patricia stop cooking. He warned that the energy of her agitation was going into the food she prepared, and we were then ingesting that agitation. The concept of not cooking was difficult for Patricia. We still could not eat most restaurant food. We bought a lot of take-out meals from the local natural grocery store and took them to Walden Pond, where we ate and then plunged into the water to cool off.

The Friday following the healing workshop, Patricia had a bodywork session with Kristine Schares, another resident of the Greenwood House. Kristine gave Patricia insights into changes her body was undergoing. For the previous two months, Patricia had found herself repeatedly scratching her shoulders and feeling an indentation in them like bra-strap marks of a woman with pendulous breasts. She could see the depressions in her skin when she looked in the mirror. Patricia, however, had small breasts and never wore a bra. When Patricia mentioned these marks, Kristine replied that was her harness. Kristine had seen harnesses before and told Patricia that now that hers was surfacing, she would be able to release it. Over the next few weeks, the marks first became more prominent, then gradually disappeared. Patricia and I both became intrigued with the process of looking at the body as a metaphor for our emotions. The more we were willing to do so, the more intriguing the process became.

The second week in May we began house hunting in earnest. Every Tuesday and Thursday morning I drove into the country and bought local papers in hopes of finding what we wanted. On Sundays we bought the *Boston Globe* as early as possible and called any ads for house rentals which seemed good prospects. Our desire to avoid new carpet, recent renovations, and gas heat ruled out many places right away. Many others indicated pets were not allowed.

The rentals we did look at all had problems that made them unsuitable for us. A converted cider mill in Holliston had lovely surroundings but was too moldy. A three-bedroom house in Natick was beautifully maintained but too close to major highways. When it became clear we were having trouble finding a house that met our needs, we looked at apartments. A three-bedroom apartment in Wellesley had possibilities, but we decided its old-fashioned gas stove and peeling paint would be too hazardous.

As June neared, pressure mounted to find a house before summer heat scorched the Boston area. All our spare time was spent in the search. Memorial Day weekend we thought we had found a place in Wellesley. The grey colonial's exterior looked run down, but the inside was in fairly good condition. After oscillating between fears of making another wrong choice like we had in Great Barrington and our urgent need to get out of the city before summer, we chose to listen to our intuition. We decided this was not a good place for us and withdrew our application.

The critical importance of moving was underscored on June seventeenth when my Watertown landlord, Glen, installed new carpet in the apartment next door. Carpet fumes filled the hallway and entered our apartment, bringing on muscle aching, irritability, and confusion. I called Glen and asked him to open windows in the other apartment to air out the fumes. He agreed but then opened the windows only a couple of inches.

This latest crisis pushed us to become creative with various resources we had acquired. Doing meta-integration exercises, advanced energy-balancing techniques developed by Steven Rochlitz, gave temporary relief. New autodetox remedies helped our bodies eliminate toxins, but we needed to figure out what to do about the carpet fumes themselves. We visualized filling our apartment and the newly carpeted one with MariEL energy. This helped but not enough. The most effective tool turned out to be the Tibetan purification chant, which Patricia had learned from Sheila.

The first evening after the carpet was installed, we did the chant in the living room where Patricia slept. Although the living room opened into the hallway and had direct exposure to carpet fumes, Patricia felt minimal effects from them and awoke the next morning feeling relatively well. We failed to do the chant in the bedroom where I slept. I woke up with muscle aching and other carpet-related symptoms. To our amazement doing the chant in that room led to clearing of the chemical smell and to relief of my symptoms.

We were grateful for the resources we had to bring to bear on this latest chemical exposure but wanted out of the apartment and out of the city. We further intensified our search. I spoke with John, the property manager for the company which owned the Greenwood House. He agreed to show us a house down the street from our friends. We made the now-familiar trip to Sharon with much anticipation about finding a place in the country near people who had helped in our healing. The house was a cozy two-bedroom Cape surrounded by conservation land. Although the house was two hundred years old, it was well-maintained. In fact, too well-maintained for our chemical sensitivities. Rooms on the first floor had just been painted and the hardwood floors were recently polyurethaned. The forced hot air by oil heat was also contraindicated for someone with environmental illness.

Patricia and I had markedly different responses to this house. I developed symptoms which led me to conclude it would not work for us. Patricia felt wonderful and was excited by feeling clear-headed and symptom-free despite the paint and polyurethane. She reflected on her past experiences looking at houses and apartments during twelve moves in the last thirteen years. While looking at them, she always felt spacy and had difficulty thinking. Her experience in this house was profoundly different, and she knew she wanted to live in it. Patricia did not know what to do with the anger and disappointment she felt when I called John, telling him we were not interested in this house but wanted to be called if others became available.

More than ever, we wanted to find a place where we could live. On July second I had another session with Helios, channeled by Sheila Simon. When I told him about the latest developments in our housing search, his reply shocked me. He asked what I would say if he told me we could live in any of the places we had looked at. I was speechless. He added that in looking at them and being confronted with the fears they stimulated, Patricia and I had been working on the core issue of our illness—disconnection from the physical. He said that in order to move beyond the current impasse we would have to give up old beliefs that no longer supported us.

Helios reminded me to choose our next house because we wanted to live there rather than to avoid toxins. He said the Sharon house would be a good place for us. It was time to stop running around, time to choose a place to move in and ground the energy. He said that all the activity we had engaged in was merely a way to disperse the energy and avoid really "getting here." After informing me that every dwelling has an angel overseeing it, Helios suggested we sit outside the house and pray to its angel for assistance. If we approached the house with love and a belief that it would support us and could not harm us, then it would be a healthy place for us. Helios warned that if we thought the house would hurt us, we would suffer many afflictions. Regarding the polyurethane, he said it would be manageable because the warm weather would allow us to keep windows open and keep fresh air flowing through the house.

Following the session, I walked to the house we had looked at, named the "Curran House" after its original owners. As I sat on the lawn, I knew I wanted to live there too. In many ways it was what Patricia and I were looking for. It had become clear that no place would meet all our requirements for safety. We were learning we could not find safety outside ourselves. When I meditated on the angel of the house, I felt a pair of large wings enfold me and was given the impression things would somehow work out.

I called Patricia and briefed her on the session and my visit to the house. She thanked the house angel for keeping the house available for us while I came to my senses. As I called John to tell him about our decision to live there, I felt not only my enthusiasm but also my fears, fears about how we would cope with the chemicals, the heating system, and any other problems that might arise. And I remembered Helios' admonition to focus on how the house would support us. To do so and to be well, we would have to deal with our fears not only about the house but about being fully alive on the Earth.

# CHAPTER TWELVE

# Confronting Fears

For five days after telling John we wanted the Curran House, we anxiously awaited approval of our rental application. Its arrival on July seventh began the next phase in our healing. We had to commit ourselves to living there. We wanted to but had no idea how we would do it. Helios and Vywamus, as teachers from subtle realms, could make suggestions, but Patricia and I were the ones who had to implement them in our daily lives. With our current financial situation, renting the Sharon house meant giving up the Watertown apartment, our backup during the failed move to Great Barrington. If this house did not work out, we would have no place to fall back on. Patricia reminded me we needed to focus on what we wanted, not on what we were afraid of. Over the next six months, we would encounter numerous situations which stimulated our fears. Repeatedly, we had to choose between being dominated by them and surmounting them.

On July eighth Patricia consulted Helios through Sheila Simon for more advice about how to succeed in the new house. He told her to relax and stay focused in the present. He suggested we continue to get frequent bodywork sessions, utilize the support of the healing group in Sharon, and talk with Vywamus often. When Patricia asked about the angel of the house, Helios responded that she had a feminine energy and worked with a beautiful rose-colored light. We could receive her support by allowing the rose color to embrace us and ground us.

Patricia also inquired about the best way to deal with any reactions to chemicals from recent renovations in the Sharon house and to our possessions from Great Barrington. Helios said that with the continuing influx of creative energy, we could easily clear and reenergize things. He encouraged us to be innovative with what we had learned. For example, we could use the MariEL energy grids to clear our possessions and the new house of adverse chemicals and energies. Other techniques he recommended for clearing included burning sage and surrounding things with white light.

By Thursday, July ninth, I was ready to make the leap from the "known" of the Watertown apartment where I had lived for fourteen years to the "unknown" of the house in Sharon with its fresh coats of paint and polyurethane. I wrote my landlord a letter giving him notice I would vacate my apartment by August fifteenth. I let myself feel the fear that this venture stirred up in me. I was determined to move ahead and leave my sensitivities behind.

That evening I also wrote a letter resigning from my position as medical director of the child-guidance center where I had worked for thirteen years. In recent weeks I had again started feeling fatigued and drowsy there. At first I worried that these symptoms reflected worsening of my mold sensitivities, but muscle testing and discussion with Michael indicated they were a message from my body saying it was time to leave the center as well. Michael, through Mary Jonaitis, said that in the course of my healing, my body's energies had accelerated and it was getting to be time to do something different. Now when I went to work at the guidance center, I had to step down my energies and experienced this as drowsiness and fatigue.

Thoughts of leaving the guidance center generated more anxiety. Part of me knew I needed to move on, but it had been my primary source of income for thirteen years. Working there half-time had offered me a regular income and flexibility to pursue other interests. Under Governor William Weld, the atmosphere had changed as the state's mental health system was dismantled. Funding for the guidance center had been cut drastically. While there were four psychiatrists when I started, I was now the only one left. I faced constant pressure to do more and to do it quicker.

Resigning would give me time to help others with immune dysfunction and also to write about our healing. However, I was uncertain about how well I would do if I needed to work in another job setting.

The next day we picked up keys for the Curran House and spent a couple of hours there. We were thrilled to find that the smells of fresh paint and polyurethane did not produce intense reactions as they had a year and a half earlier.

That afternoon I phoned my boss, Rick, at the guidance center, and arranged to meet with him the next day. Although I did not tell him I planned to resign, my heart pounded throughout our brief conversation. After I hung up, an inner voice reassured me by saying, "You are here with a gift of healing and it's time to express it." Leaving my job would be a step in that direction.

When I went to talk with Rick, our interaction removed any remaining doubts I had about the wisdom of resigning. His first response upon seeing me was to make sure I would not take more than a half-hour credit for quality review work I had done that week. The guidance center had reduced the time in my schedule for that task from the three hours per week listed in my contract to a half hour without reducing the workload.

Rick seemed surprised by my resignation. Since I had worked at the guidance center for thirteen years, my presence had come to be taken for granted. I framed my departure in terms of my desire to pursue other ventures. By the time the meeting ended, I felt like a great weight had been lifted. I looked forward to being free from that job in another month.

The following week we did the bulk of our moving. We hired a company called The Marakesh Express to move large items from storage in Waltham to Sharon. These were things which were in the moldy Great Barrington house for eighteen months before spending the last three months in storage. We were uncertain about their safety for us and had most of them put in the garage until we could sort through them. We rented a medium-sized truck and moved our beds and other large items from Watertown ourselves.

Then we started sleeping in Sharon. We kept the windows wide open to minimize reactions to paint and polyurethane. Any reactions which did occur were relatively short-lived. We now recognized that our bodies' symptoms were not always from the toxic effects of chemicals. Sometimes the reactions were our bodies' efforts to clear something, part of our healing. When I developed crampy abdominal pain, we identified it as a clearing of paint symptoms which first emerged during the shellac debacle in Great Barrington. I worked through it by using my breath and grounding my energy. Thereafter, I had no more of those symptoms.

Other emotions besides fear also came up for us. On July twenty-fourth we went to a workshop with Vywamus, this time channeled by Sheila Simon, on healing the feminine. The goal was greater integration of the masculine and feminine. Sixteen women attended. I was the only man. My task was to sit at the front of the room and receive whatever rage the women held toward the masculine as they stood before me, one at a time, and expressed it. I was relieved that Vywamus placed a protective energetic shield around me so that as the anger came at me, I wasn't penetrated by it. Even with the shield, the demonstrations of rage deeply affected me. I was moved by how much abuse these women, individually and collectively, had suffered.

When it was Patricia's turn, she felt a tube of energy surround her. Vywamus asked her to express through her body what she was feeling. She began by crouching in a little ball on the floor and then proceeded to deal with her father's abusive treatment of her by screaming at me as if I were he. She raged about the beatings with a belt, her fear of speaking, and the fact that she grew up feeling she was not allowed to move, not allowed to breathe, not really allowed to exist. She felt these words coming up from her belly and out of her mouth without her mind being involved at all. She now understood what Vywamus meant when he spoke of emotions being stored in the body.

After venting her emotions, Patricia was asked by Vywamus to again express with her body how she felt. She unfolded like a flower and did a full backward bend touching her hands to the floor, something she had never been able to do before in her life. She thought for days afterward about what a significant role unexpressed emotions had played in limiting her movement.

Following the workshop, we returned to trying to get our lives back in order. As we finished packing up the apartment, I said good-bye to what had been my home for the last fourteen years. While checking out an office in Worcester to do psychiatric consultations, I was not troubled by chemical smells as I had been when I rented in the same building two years before. I was pleased and relieved that I did not react to chemicals and perfumes in the copy shop as I had only two months earlier.

In August, we bought organic cotton sheets and were able to use them after five washings. That we could use them at all was a momentous event after being unable to use new sheets or clothes no matter how many times we washed them. For the first time in six months, I slept with sheets on my bed. Never would I have imagined I would take such pleasure in what is for most people an everyday occurrence.

Not everything went smoothly. We both continued to have itchy, red rashes over much of our bodies below the neck. The itching was so intense sometimes that we could not do anything else. Our best assessment was that the itching was related to releasing rage, as Helios suggested. We followed his advice to take cold showers, eat cooling foods, avoid hot, spicy foods, and lightly rub our skin rather than scratch it. At times we felt achy, feverish, and fatigued, like we were coming down with the flu, but it never developed. When Patricia started to feel achy and sluggish at the holistic physicians' office where she worked, she took it as a sign that she, too, should leave her job soon.

There were more and more indications that we were moving beyond the devastation environmental illness had caused us. In early September we went shopping for underwear and other clothes. Although we smelled chemicals in the store, our reactions were minimal. By the time we returned home, Patricia felt achy and tired, but her symptoms went away after a half-hour nap in the Bio-tron Projector. Having new underwear to replace that which had been slowly falling apart was another step back toward normality. We were able to wear it after a couple of washings.

The gains we had made also manifested in work settings. I resumed doing psychiatric consultations at the Brookline office where a mold smell had previously caused me to feel achy and nauseous. Now the smell didn't bother me, and I could work without an air filter.

Along with these improvements, we faced challenges. We noticed a strange smell in the house's basement and tried to determine whether it was from mold or chemicals. We wanted to avoid repeating the basement quagmire which forced us out of Great Barrington. The several experts I had assess the problem each gave a different opinion. One said the furnace should be replaced, because it was too old. Another noticed dark stains on boards next to the stairs suggesting there had been a fire. When I asked John, the property manager, he said ten years earlier a fire caused by lightning destroyed a barn which had been next to the house. Patricia and I were furious that despite our specific questions about any major problems in the house, we had not been informed of this important piece of information before we signed the lease.

We considered a range of options to eliminate the sickening odor which emanated from the first-floor heating vents. We decided the least complicated initial step would be to put a dehumidifier in the basement. Drying the basement led to a marked reduction in the smell. Aware that there probably was a lot of dust and debris in the heating system, we decided that having it cleaned would further reduce the odor.

This event turned out to be one more occasion to confront our fears. After researching various options, we hired a local company to do the job. The cleaning itself was benign, just vacuuming the ducts. Then we had to decide whether to have a disinfectant sprayed for the purpose of eliminating mold and dust mites. We debated fervently about what to do. Given that mold caused such a problem in the last house and that forced hot air would blow dust around, we opted for the spraying. At the same time we worried about the chemicals in the spray and feared they might force us to leave this house too.

When we turned the heat on after the spraying, we felt achy and cloudy-headed. Patricia became panicky, and we decided to go for a walk in the woods. During the walk Patricia experienced a sudden, dramatic change in how her head felt. She noticed a tremendous lightening of the energy around her head as if layers were quickly falling away. A voice in her head told her she had just opened to her channel. She thought about how this happened after she chose to confront and stay present with her fears about the chemicals sprayed in the heating system. By using the tools we had for clearing reactions, we were able to lessen our symptoms, which went away over the next two days, never to return in response to the heat being turned on.

In mid-September I had an hour reading with Michael, channeled by Mary Jonaitis. It was an opportunity to get another perspective on the process Patricia and I were going through. Michael said that our nervous systems were significantly stronger. We talked about the healing process and my plans to write this book. I noted that in what would be the middle section of the book, we recognized the possibility of getting better. Michael replied that was a critical point. Unless the belief systems open to believe it is possible to heal, the deep, internal process that is needed cannot occur.

As we discussed other topics, Michael stressed the importance of people getting to their true feelings if they are to overcome their disease, whatever it may be. We had heard this said many times in many ways but were still unsure about how to do it. Michael said these feelings could be accessed through acknowledging and allowing the inner child's presence. He described different systems of inner child work. I most liked one which he said came from the native Hawaiian tradition of Ho'oponopono.

In Ho'oponopono the whole person is said to be made of the mother-self, the father-self, and the child-self. The father-self is the bringer of awareness of the skies, of thoughts, of how to be in the world of creativity and ideas. The mother-self teaches how to be in the body and on the physical plane. The child-self is that which is spirit and connects to inspiration. Without the child-self, one cannot have inspiration. Without inspiration, or being in spirit, there is not much enthusiasm for life and one feels like a victim. Michael added that then a variety of illnesses could occur.

Michael said prior to my illness my father-self was rather well developed, but my mother-self was quite undeveloped. In addition, my child-self was only partly heard because the child-self can only come in fully when father and mother are both present. Only half of the spirit was available to me, because without the grounding effect of the mother-self, I could not hold the full vibration of spirit. Michael described Ho'oponopono as extending into complete forgiveness. With forgiveness comes detachment so that one can feel one's full freedom.

He emphasized the importance of individuals' personal quests to find their truth, to be as big as they really are, and to let go of victimization. He saw victimization as being at the base of both environmental illness and chronic fatigue syndrome. At the psychic emotional level the victimization had to be broken off. Michael closed by commending Patricia and me for our success thus far in what had been an extremely difficult passage through our illness.

Around that time, there was growing media coverage of Persian Gulf War veterans, who complained of a wide range of health problems similar to those seen in environmental illness and chronic fatigue syndrome. A National Public Radio report highlighted petrochemical poisoning as the possible basis of symptoms including joint aching, fatigue, and sensitivity to low levels of chemicals. The descriptions by several veterans at a congressional hearing held in Boston on September twentieth underscored how much their lives had been disrupted by unexplained symptoms which developed after they served in the Gulf.

While I did not work directly with any Gulf War veterans, I did start working with a number of people with environmental illness and chronic fatigue syndrome. Some came to classes on energy balancing which Patricia and I taught; others came for individual sessions. Generally we began with the Rochlitz exercises which helped lessen sensitivities and increase energy. The focus in the individual sessions varied from doing advanced energy balancing to identifying and clearing emotional issues which hampered immune functioning.

A variety of themes emerged. Some clients had feelings of powerlessness and a need to please others, regardless of the cost to themselves. Several dated the onset of their sensitivities to involvement in a car accident. Whether initiated by a sudden event or long-standing patterns, a common underlying theme was a sense of loss of control and inability to determine the events of one's life.

Patricia and I found that daily events forced us to confront unresolved feelings we still held. When Patricia's friend, Jackie, was diagnosed as having scabies, Patricia and I both feared that we might also be affected. Tiny vesicular lesions had been appearing on my hands for several months, but we had associated them with our rashes and attributed them to the clearing process we were going through. To get a professional opinion, I consulted a dermatologist. Although the skin scraping he did was negative for scabies, he recommended treatment with Kwell lotion to be safe.

For me, mentioning Kwell and being safe in the same breath was an oxymoron. Kwell contained a strong parasiticide with neurotoxic effects. When we had tried a more natural solution to the flea problem two years earlier, it nearly killed me. We decided to go ahead with this treatment for a couple reasons. Jackie thought she had gotten the scabies from a cat, and we wanted to make sure Patricia's cats did not become infected with scabies as had happened with the fleas. Also, our testing indicated that using the Kwell would help Patricia clear previous exposures to pesticides.

We showered and then spread the Kwell over our bodies from the neck down. It had to stay on for twelve hours. I reacted with transient knee pain but had no other symptoms. Patricia became fatigued, achy, depressed, and tearful, which we assumed was secondary to the neurotoxic effects of the lotion. Nine hours in the Bio-Tron Projector helped reverse the Kwell's effects. The next day Patricia washed her cats with the shampoo which two years before produced neuromuscular incoordination in me when I was three rooms away from her. I now remained symptom-free except for transient nausea. The shampoo bothered Patricia, but her symptoms cleared in a few hours.

Although we survived the Kwell application, we continued itching. The source of our exasperating rashes became clear to us after Sheila and Vywamus provoked Patricia in a class one evening, stirring up her rage as Andy Cappanigro had done with me six months earlier. When we returned home, Patricia stormed up to her room and sat on the floor crying, screaming, and pounding her fists on the floor. This torrent of uncontrolled anger frightened me, and I tried to calm her down. After I gave her some Rescue Remedy, a Bach flower remedy used in crisis situations, Patricia stopped crying and screaming but resumed scratching. She cursed at me and said I should have let her scream. Over the next few months, the rash and itching slowly faded away.

While our lives were improving, we also had many frustrations to cope with. Shortly after the Kwell experience, Patricia bounced her third check in a week. At first I responded by putting more money in her bank account and paying her Visa bill. Throughout that day I became increasingly angry and depressed until by evening, in what was for me unusual behavior, my anger erupted. I roamed the house looking for a way to express the rage which was insistent on busting out. I began by ripping a stack of telephone books into pieces. Next, I smashed wine glasses into the fireplace in the den, but still more was ready to explode. Finally, an inner voice told me to go into the garage where I used a hammer to demolish a wooden chair.

Patricia watched this destruction with fear and fascination. She remembered how Adriana helped her move some of her anger during a bodywork session. Adriana had emphasized the importance of having someone present while you let the anger out. Patricia's father had smashed several of his favorite chairs in a fit of rage over her delinquent behavior when she was a teenager. Patricia had to work hard to stay present for me and for herself as I destroyed the chair in the garage. The experience of watching me changed our relationship in profound ways. Patricia learned she could stay present with me while I was raging and not get beaten or killed. She began to feel safer in my presence. She said I should get angry more often, because she could see that my aura was stronger. I did feel more energized and more present in my body.

As we passed through layer after layer of sensitivities and fears, new ones kept emerging, but there were indications something was shifting, something was changing inside us that reflected an opening to parts of ourselves we had not been in touch with before. In late October while walking in the woods near our house, I sensed a lightness in my body. I noticed the bright green mold coating many trees after three days of rain and experienced it as something beautiful to enjoy looking at rather than to make me sick as it had the year before.

Three days later, I had my own opening of connection to higher self, even more striking than Patricia's a month earlier. While we were talking in the dining room, I suddenly became aware of intense light and heat in the room and inside me. Then the area above and around my head opened, and I had the sense of more space. My body began to move like I was wriggling my way out of a cocoon. When I was finally free, the heat and light slowly faded away. I was left feeling more fully present in my body and more grounded. Patricia had not perceived the heat or light but laughed with delight as she recognized my movements to be like those of a butterfly setting itself free. She felt different in my presence, more energetic, more clearheaded, and more grounded. We were enchanted to see that the chemical sensitivities which had shattered our lives had also opened a door which allowed us to experience new parts of ourselves.

As I worked with more chemically sensitive people, I noted another common thread among many of them—that of having grown up in abusive families. The severity of abuse varied and the level of abuse did not seem to be an indicator of the degree of illness. However, a number of patients described the onset of their symptoms as starting during therapy that uncovered or examined their abuse histories.

Patricia recalled that her sensitivities intensified when her psychotherapy shifted from her father's behavior to aspects of her relationship with her mother. Her therapist pushed her to look at how her mother had allowed the abuse and was abusive herself. Her therapist told her she had created a false image of her mother in order to have an illusion of safety. Patricia had not allowed herself to be aware of her true feelings as a child. This therapy went on prior to our move to Great Barrington, a time during which Patricia became much sicker. She abruptly stopped the therapy when we moved.

A discussion with Michael on this subject revealed his understanding that when a victim of abuse has no way to process those experiences, the memories of the abuse get pushed deeply into the body. When that person engages in psychotherapy and the memories are brought to the surface, they need a way to move out of the physical body. Possible avenues include expressive movement, the visual arts, or bodywork. When the energy of these memories is stirred up but not released, the experience of abuse is literally stuck in the body, roaming around causing illness. This view was similar to Vywamus' explanation that the body reflects or mirrors back to a person unexpressed emotion. Vywamus also talked about the necessity of clearing belief patterns associated with abuse so that the abused individual can live in his or her power in the present and let go of the past.

Some of the clearing Patricia and I were doing involved more recent traumas. On November tenth we drove three hours to Brewster, New York, so that I could attend a one-day class with Steven Rochlitz on "Science and Healing." The trip brought back memories of our many trips to Great Barrington. In Brewster we stayed at the same motel I had fled two years earlier because of its mold smell. This time we noticed the smell but were able to stay there using our own linen. The next morning we cleared the muscle aching we had by listening to Tibetan overtone chanting tapes and using the Bio-Tron Projector.

Steven's class included information on kinesiology, physics, and biology as related to healing. Of particular interest, given our recent work using sound, were his comments that restoring health involves restoring an organ or system to its own natural resonant frequency. Various factors, such as drugs, sugar, Candida, and psychological trauma, cause imbalance in the body and lead to disease. Steven taught a variety of techniques that balanced the body's energies and accessed the body's wisdom, so as to learn which action, among a variety of options, would optimally assist the body to vibrate at its own resonant frequency.

The next weekend, Patricia and I attended the second level of Ethel Lombardi's MariEL training. Ethel told us how the vibratory rate of the Earth continued to increase on a daily basis. Everyone was attempting to integrate the new frequency and, in the process, different physical symptoms could arise, including muscle aching or spasms. She said that many people were panicking because they wanted to go back to the way things were before, but it was not possible to go back. She showed us different techniques to allow us to align with and ground the new energies and to facilitate a clearing of memories. Ethel emphasized the powerful negative effects of the thought pattern of not wanting to be here. The alternative was to acknowledge this thought and then choose to be fully present.

By that time I had begun writing this book and would read chapters to Patricia as she worked in the kitchen. She always said she wanted to hear what I had written but often became agitated and even abusive toward me when I did. Then she would feel terrible, physically and emotionally. It would take two or three days for her to feel better. After this happened several times, we realized that she was feeling the same as she had in Great Barrington, cloudy-headed and flulike, with aching down to her bones.

Quite by accident, or perhaps guided by her soul, she had a

remarkable insight the fourth time this scenario repeated itself. After I finished reading to her, she turned on some music and started dancing in the kitchen. When she stopped, her bones no longer hurt. The aching Patricia had been feeling in the core of her body had moved out of the bones and was now in the muscles. Over the next four hours she felt the pain move out completely, first from the deep muscles, then from the superficial muscles, and then her skin ached and was sore to the touch as it often had been when she was a child. Finally, she found herself moving as if she were in pain, but the pain was completely gone. She realized all that was left was the thoughtform, and she chose to let it go. These experiences led her to begin studying movement as a vehicle for self-healing.

While we did much of our clearing work at home, it went on outside as well. In late November, I took a train to New York City to spend a day with my friend Les. The trip brought up many fears. Since becoming sick, I had not done any extensive train travel. I worried about how well I would feel being enclosed in the train for five hours. I also worried about tolerating the hotel room and what I would eat. I took water, a small air filter, and some food with me but left my sheets at home. I decided to use the hotel's.

On the train, I initially smelled a chemical odor that made my muscles ache, but within an hour the smell abated and I felt better. When Les met me at Penn Station, he commented that I continued to look healthier. We went to a hotel near Lincoln Center. The hotel room was attractively decorated, not too smelly, and had windows that opened. The sheets on my bed were polyester. The pillow was foam rubber. I did a meditation to release whatever energetic blocks might keep me from feeling comfortable and resolved that I would be all right.

After eating dinner at a nearby Thai restaurant, we went to a performance of the New York City Ballet. Les frequently attended such events. For me, going to the ballet had been rare before my environmental illness and impossible once I became sick. The crowds of people with perfumes, hair sprays, and other smelly personal-care products would have been too much for my fragile immune system.

The people seated around me that evening offered a sample of what previously would have made me ill. In front of me was a young woman who smelled as if she had splashed perfume all over herself. To the left was an older women whose strong perfume was complemented by the mothball smell on her wool sweater, which had probably just come out of storage. Despite being surrounded by these chemicals, I had only the slightest symptoms and enjoyed the performance. That night I slept in the hotel room without difficulty.

On Sunday I took the train back to Sharon and resumed writing this book. I was writing about the events of February 1991, when we could stay at neither place we were renting because of the shellac exposure at the Red House. Both Patricia and I began to reexperience the extreme muscle cramping, pain, and fatigue we had back then. Patricia was affected physically much more than I was. She said she felt like she had when she lived in her roach–spray–contaminated apartment in Brookline. She recalled the image of surviving a nuclear disaster. Recognizing the recurrence of symptoms as part of a clearing of the shellac poisoning, we used muscle testing to find out what would facilitate the process. Toning, movement, being in the Bio-Tron Projector, and listening to Tibetan chanting tapes helped with the clearing, which continued for several days.

In light of the distress my writing was causing Patricia, I considered taking a day off. When I mentioned that idea to her, she insisted the writing continue and asked me to hurry up. She hoped that when I finished the section on our worst days in Great Barrington, she would start to feel better.

I reviewed with her the events of March to August 1991 when we started on the macrobiotic diet and had to sleep in a tent. Her shoulders and back again became extremely tight, her whole rib cage ached, and her cloudy-headedness returned. We wondered why she had such a strong reaction to what I wrote about and used her recurrence of symptoms to study the healing process. Some days we spent hours muscle testing to understand what was behind her symptoms and what would help.

The night before Christmas, Patricia's healing took an unexpected turn. She had felt achy throughout the day. While cooking dinner, she became angry and depressed about it being Christmas, having no money to buy presents, but feeling like she had to. She remembered her childhood and how frustrated her mother always was at Christmas, buying gifts for six children and feeling she could not afford them. Recalling Helios' warning to be aware of the energy she put into the food she cooked, Patricia tried to focus on joy and peace. At the same time, without recognizing what she was doing, Patricia was attempting to suppress feelings of helplessness, hopelessness, and rage that were bubbling up inside her. When she finally sat down to eat, she was unable to contain those feelings any longer. Sobbing, she jumped up from the table, ran outside, and collapsed on the frozen ground.

As Patricia lay there, feeling out of control, she closed her eyes and saw thousands of black dots. She had one flashback after another of dinnertime scenes from her childhood, of her father yelling at her and the other children, pushing their faces into their food, screaming at them, and beating them with his belt. The more she thought about those memories, the more hysterical and out-of-control she became. When she was too cold, she came inside, draped herself over the washing machine, and continued to cry, feeling like a child who had just been beaten. Finally, she went to bed for a long, deep sleep.

The next morning after eating, Patricia felt exhausted and her stomach hurt. Again she lay on the ground to clear memories of her father and mealtime. When she thought of the many black dots she had seen the night before, she remembered Ethel Lombardi saying that the black dots were negative thoughtforms. When she came back in the house and told me about this, I realized that the little child in Patricia felt so traumatized by mealtime at her house that it was not safe for her to eat. For the next two days, she went outside after each meal and lay on the ground to release whatever memories came up. She facilitated the release through toning, movement, and, at times, screaming. As she lay on the ground, she could feel energy leaving her belly and flowing into the Earth.

Although it was winter, Patricia did not feel cold outside. However, during the releasing process she began shivering deep within. The first two times when the shaking started, she came inside, thinking she needed to get out of the cold. When she did that, she developed tremendous pain in the area of her kidneys. The third time she realized she should let the pain go. She lay on her back and visualized the energy of fear flowing from her kidneys into the Earth. Within a minute, the pain was gone and she stopped shaking.

On the third day, the clearing process intensified. In the morning Patricia spent more than an hour outside on the ground releasing cellular memories. She wanted to come in earlier but followed the direction of her body to continue releasing. When she finally did come in, muscle testing indicated she had released a major portion of the trauma which had been locked in her belly. During a final session that evening, she saw a lightning bolt with her inner vision and heard an inner voice say it was safe to eat now. Our minds did not fully comprehend what had happened, but thereafter Patricia gradually reintroduced many previously restricted foods to her diet without adverse reactions.

All the releasing Patricia and I were doing seemed most opportune as we completed 1992 and prepared to begin 1993. On December thirty-first we heard Steven McFadden, author of *Ancient Voices, Current Affairs*, on a local radio show. He talked about the Harmonic Convergence of 1987 as indicating the end of a 24,000-year cycle and the beginning of a twenty-five-year period of purification, a time of clearing the way for higher-vibrational energies that already were coming to the Earth. Change was occurring at all levels of society, including major restructuring of businesses and governments, to allow spirit to express more fully in the physical.

Hearing Steven McFadden helped us put our battles with environmental illness in a broader perspective. On one level, our extreme sensitivities reflected an imbalance in the world where toxic chemicals had been developed and used without awareness or concern about their impact on the Earth and her inhabitants. On another level, our illness was our personal wake-up call to look at areas in our lives where we were not being fully present. To heal the illness at its core would require a deep restructuring of our lives on all levels. We cried tears of joy as we acknowledged we had already started this process which we did not understand and which was beyond our control.

# CHAPTER THIRTEEN

# Freedom from the Inside Out

Over the next six months our process continued with an emphasis on healing the inner origins of our sensitivities. Patricia had become acutely aware that what was helping us was radically different from what was offered in the holistic physicians' office where she worked. She felt there was such a conflict in the approaches that she needed to leave that environment to more fully explore the path we were on. Having given several months' notice, she left that position on December 30, 1992, and planned to get a part-time job as a visiting nurse. She thought this change would free up her energies to move in a new direction. Instead, she plunged into a paralyzing depression.

Throughout January, Patricia awakened each day planning to get ready and go job hunting, but by midway through breakfast she would be sobbing and telling me she hurt all over and could not do anything. She would drag herself back to bed, filled with shame about her inability to pull herself together. She had been depressed in the past but never had experienced such a devastating level of dysfunction. Nothing she nor we did helped. She did not share with me her fear that I would leave her because she was not meeting her obligations in our partnership.

At a loss for what to do, she sought advice from Vywamus, through Sheila Simon. He gently told her she was okay, that she was grieving and should allow the process to continue. He said I had provided her with a safe environment in which she could experience her emotions and that this would lead to a greater level of creativity for both of us. He added that we were touching into the purpose of the masculine and feminine in relationship and should not fear what was happening.

Despite these assurances, we were deeply troubled by Patricia's ongoing malaise, depression, and fatigue. Although most of her physical symptoms were ones she, for years, had related to chemical sensitivities, now we were determined to heal the problem at its core rather than by looking for an external explanation. Taking a cue from Vywamus, we began an in-depth study of the impact our thoughts and emotions had on our health.

One day when Patricia became incredibly tired after only a short walk, we used muscle testing to help us understand the inner dynamics which had brought on her exhaustion. We were guided to focus on her thoughts right before the onset of the fatigue. She had been thinking about attending a CPR training which would be required for any new nursing job she might take. She hated CPR trainings and the memories they evoked of many stressful, traumatic experiences during cardiac resuscitations in the coronary care units where she had worked for so many years. After she visualized releasing those memories while lying on the ground in our yard, she felt lighter and her cheeks were flushed with color. She also felt clear-headed and energized.

When I tried to let myself feel my emotions, I was aware of little, at first; but with my intention to experience them, anger, frustration, sadness, and rage surfaced. Once the process of focusing on my emotions had begun, if I did not allow myself to feel them, situations appeared to intensify them and bring them to my awareness.

The first Thursday in January, Patricia gave a presentation at the Greenwood House on movement and healing. I planned to support her by attending. However, when the time came, I was too depressed to go. Something inside me needed to shift. I felt like either it was going to change or I was going to die. After trudging a mile and a half through foot-deep snow, I came to a rocky ledge and flung myself down on a large, flat rock. Lying there on my back, I did not know what to do, but an inner voice directed me to release self-hatred, grief, and other judgments and repressed emotions I was holding inside. When I closed my eyes and integrated several meditations I had been working with, I was surprised to see the colors of the chakras vibrating in my energy field. I felt renewed and refreshed and was aware of an expansion and a flowing of my energy.

As I walked home, I wondered why this experience happened on this particular day. Then I realized the next day marked exactly one year since my first session with Vywamus. The work with him had accelerated our healing process. I honored this latest clearing as part of completing that one-year cycle and preparing for the next.

One support for us, as we chose to leave the past behind and move on to a new definition of ourselves and our lives, was a weekly class with Vywamus and Sheila. Vywamus described 1993 as the year of opening the heart to be able to love self and others. He said that when the heart is closed, people tend to collapse on themselves, which manifests as depression, feelings of victimization, or physical exhaustion. We worked with grounding our energy, toning, movement, meditations, and experiential exercises to expand the heart and integrate what Vywamus described as waves of higher vibrational energy which were coming to the Earth.

Around the times Vywamus said an influx of energy occurred, we often felt tired or developed physical symptoms such as headaches, muscle aching, or even a cold. He told us these symptoms were part of the body's attempts to adjust to the new energy. A number of my patients had similar symptoms at those times and attributed them to having the flu. Patricia and I wondered whether they, too, were experiencing the effects of the higher-vibrational energy. We also speculated about the possible connection between this energy and the growing number of people with environmental illness and chronic fatigue syndrome.

Merely releasing self-defeating thoughts or feeling our emotions often was not sufficient to produce a change. Sometimes we needed to go more deeply into our psyches. The day after a beautiful class with Vywamus, Patricia awoke feeling exhausted and achy as if she had been beaten up. When she asked in a meditation why she had such a hard time opening her heart, she received the image of having been battered as an infant.

Deeply disturbed by this image, she spoke with Vywamus about it. He explained to her that it did not matter if the image was of a real event or not. The important thing was to acknowledge her frightened inner child and to work with her. He said there was no need to go in and retrieve every single memory of abuse in this or other lifetimes. He added that, in fact, she could go crazy trying to do so. He suggested she simply focus on acknowledging she was clearing memories of abuse and allow them to release from her body.

Vywamus recommended that when physical symptoms appeared, Patricia should dialogue with her inner child and critical parent and allow them to express themselves. He explained that they were trying to protect her from harm and she should thank them for expressing their concerns. She should then reassure them that everything was all right, that she was the adult now who would protect them and make decisions for them. They should relax and play.

This conversation with Vywamus unplugged a dam for Patricia. For weeks she had frequent conversations with these inner aspects of herself sparked by episodes of pain or exhaustion. She became aware that both her inner child and critical parent would clamp onto any mention of possible danger and run it in her mind until she was exhausted.

They did this out of fear that if she did not act in a certain way, her father would punish her. For example, they were afraid to get out of bed in the morning, because someone in the house might beat them. They constantly monitored what she did, assessing if she was working hard enough. One evening Patricia's thought that the meal she prepared of soup and sandwiches was more like a lunch than dinner set off an episode of what we called "collapsing." Whenever Patricia reassured her critical parent and inner child that her father was dead and could not harm her anymore and that she would look after them, she noticed a reduction in mental chatter, a relaxing of her body, and the melting away of any physical pain she was having.

In her mind, Patricia also let her inner child and critical parent speak with both of her parents and express their feelings. At first, these inner aspects of her self cried and expressed great fear. Then they moved on to anger and rage. Eventually, came understanding and forgiveness.

Startled and frightened by the dramatic effects her thoughts and feelings had on her physical body, Patricia felt out of control. Although Vywamus often told us the energies we were calling forth would magnify everything so that we could see the effects of our thoughts, we tended to forget this helpful piece of information. In the middle of an intense experience, Patricia often wondered whether she would ever be able to heal her damaged psyche.

The things that helped her varied. For three months, she continued to dialogue with her critical parent and inner child. Significant progress was made when she followed Vywamus' suggestion to talk with them about their choice to have fear or not. After that conversation, her energy increased substantially and her episodes of physical discomfort became much less frequent. Some days, processing thoughts and feelings brought about incredible shifts. Other days no noticeable change occurred with this process and an energetic balance or the Rochlitz exercises would help. We observed that intense inner work was often followed by flare-ups in Patricia's Candida. Now she was able to tolerate herbal preparations, which helped rid her body of Candida and parasites.

This work helped us see that some sensations that we might have previously attributed to chemical reactions were, indeed, related to unexpressed feelings. Along those lines, I at first thought a sensation of heaviness in my chest was a reaction to chemicals in the heating system. Muscle testing indicated it was instead related to my inner child's grief at not having been nurtured the way he would have wanted. After I grounded my energy, chose to have my cells release the grief, and filled all the cells of my being with connection to life and to a sense of being nurtured, the heaviness went away.

As our healing continued, we were able to let go of more restrictions that we had made to cope with environmental illness. I was able to pump gasoline for my car without reacting to the fumes. We were able to turn off the air filters which had been running in our bedrooms. I found I again enjoyed the generic smell of the local department store, a smell that for two years had brought on nausea, headache, and muscle aching. I could resume writing with pens made of plastic. Patricia was able to work part-time as a visiting nurse and stopped taking the small dose of antidepressant medication she had been on.

Eventually, the intense fears of Patricia's inner child and critical parent ceased and were replaced by intermittent explosions of rage. One day while she was cooking, I walked into the kitchen and stood next to her. It was as if I had entered another reality. I looked at a Corning Ware dish filled with rice and asked if that was cooked rice. Patricia became very agitated and asked what I had said. I repeated my question several times and each time her anger mounted. By the time I finished speaking, she was in a rage, yelling and hitting me. Her behavior shocked and frightened both of us.

When Patricia finally calmed down, we sorted out what had happened. She let herself become conscious of a voice which always ran in her head, monitoring what she ate, constantly planning the next meal, and making sure she chose healthy, safe foods. She realized her critical parent had not let go of the safety structure of the rotation diet, even though she had stopped following it, and was worried that she was eating too much rice. My questions about the rice seemed odd until we realized that as I entered Patricia's energy field, I experienced her inner world and reflected back to her the obsessive thoughts she was running on an unconscious level.

Patricia's outbursts of anger became more frequent. At times she was aware of the inappropriateness of her rage and felt like she was standing outside herself, watching the ranting and raving, aware that she did not really care about whatever she was screaming about. She said she felt as if she were short-circuiting and had no control over herself. As with the depression in January 1993, these expressions of intense emotion were followed by shame and fear that I would abandon her.

When Patricia questioned Vywamus about her rampages, she was told by him they were merely a way of releasing energy. He seemed unconcerned. The outbursts continued intermittently over the next two years. Both of us gradually learned to stay connected to ourselves and each other as we moved rage or witnessed its expression. Eventually, we were able to allow it to move without intense fear and even began to laugh at ourselves in the middle of these eruptions.

While Patricia focused on letting her rage move, I began working more intensely on my fears and my doubts. The last week in March, I drove to upstate New York for advanced study with Steven Rochlitz. As I ran around the house packing for the trip, I recognized how my fear was running me and how my doubts about whether I could make the trip caused me to collapse on myself. After I made the intention to support myself, I was able to be more focused and relaxed. The trip took three-and-a-half hours, including being stuck in Hartford's afternoon rush-hour traffic. I made it through by breathing, staying centered, and grounding my energy.

When I arrived at the motel in Brewster, New York, I was given the same room I had tried sixteen months earlier. Back then, the mold smell was too much and I had had to leave. Now I smelled the mold without becoming sick. The only effect was slight muscle aching. Tears of joy overcame me in response to this latest indication of how much my health had improved. I slept there two nights without a problem. In the classes on Saturday and Sunday I focused better and relaxed more around my classmates than at any of Steven's other seminars.

Not long thereafter Patricia attended a workshop in Boston given by Lena Stevens, a Michael channel from New Mexico. One of the exercises was a Native American practice that involved journeying into a cave in the Earth to find an answer to a specific question. Following up on a suggestion from Vywamus, Patricia asked to be connected to a teacher with whom she could study movement, but she fell asleep during the exercise. When she awoke, she felt ashamed and frustrated by her inability to stay present. Lena commented that people who are working on self-deprecation often had trouble staying awake in that type of exercise. Patricia found this comment helpful as she remembered Michael had told her self-deprecation was her chief negative feature. Nevertheless, she left feeling she had missed what she was supposed to receive from the workshop.

Two days later, on the spur of the moment, Patricia joined Kristine Schares who was going to a kundalini yoga class in Millis, Massachusetts. It was taught by a substitute teacher, a beautiful woman dressed all in white, who was a member of the Sikh community. That night only three students were in attendance. The teacher, Guruatma Kaur, repeatedly asked Patricia if she knew her. Although Patricia knew they had never met, she too experienced feelings of familiarity, especially about the meditation center. The sense of familiarity was so strong that Patricia recognized this must be what she had drawn to herself in the journeying exercise the previous weekend.

She arranged a weekly, private tutorial on kundalini yoga with Guruatma Kaur. Despite the added cost, Patricia chose a private session because she often was adversely affected by other people's energy. Guruatma Kaur chose a yoga set for Patricia that she was to do every day for 120 days. She also taught her a new set at each weekly meeting. Patricia found that each day, no matter how poorly she felt at the start of her yoga routine, by the end she felt pain-free and rejuvenated.

As our healing progressed, we were able to begin acknowledging how sick we had been. When I told Patricia that someone we knew was applying for disability benefits because of environmental illness, she surmised she likely would have been on disability herself if she had not met me. She reflected on how in trying to become well she had spent every penny of the fifty thousand dollars a year she earned as a critical care nurse. She had not previously allowed herself to consider the possibility of going on disability but had images of ending up on the street as a bag lady.

Patricia recognized the importance of what Vywamus had told her months earlier about my providing a safe place where she could feel her feeling body. As her physical body gradually relaxed, she became aware that she had been holding a high level of tension for a long, long time and until recently never truly felt safe. She began to recognize that on a subconscious level she continuously ran a state of fear and realized this could be one reason for her constant exhaustion. The fatigue had kept returning in spite of meticulous attention to her diet, avoidance of sugar and caffeine, and the many other things she did to take care of herself. Now, as she processed deeply held emotions and her body relaxed, the exhaustion was leaving her.

Clearing our physical and emotional bodies had profound healing effects for both of us, but there was yet another step in the process. We were fortunate to connect with a Native American teacher-healer and to participate in pipe ceremonies and sweat lodges she offered. While we both were aware of the use of saunas for detoxification, neither of us had done so. The sweat lodges were a way to detoxify ourselves in a similar manner, but in a sacred ceremony which connected us deeply to Spirit and to Mother Earth. To our amazement, we both were able to smoke the peace pipe without difficulty. We found these ceremonies comforting, inspiring, and nurturing. They gave us a sense of coming home. Attending them greatly accelerated our healing. We further expanded our diets and even found we could eat an occasional dessert.

Our experiences with lawn care gave one more indication of our improvement. By early May it was time to start mowing the lawn, and we hired a neighbor to do the job. When he came with his gasoline-powered riding mower, we were unaffected by either the gasoline fumes or the grass cuttings. I even kept the windows open while he mowed. This event was a welcome contrast to the extreme difficulties we had with cut grass just two years earlier.

Later that month, Patricia filled in for the allergy nurse at the office where she previously worked. She saw several patients she knew from before, and each one commented on how much healthier she looked. These reflections were enormously affirming in the midst of this intense clearing process which we could neither measure nor comprehend.

Another step in our healing was retrieving things which had been in the garage since coming out of storage. After airing each item outdoors for a few hours, we muscle tested for any adverse reactions. We used our abilities as MariEL practitioners to clear them of the energy they held from the past. Many had spent over a year in the toxic environment of the Great Barrington house. Now we could tolerate them. We moved my computer, bookcases, and some clothing into the house without difficulty.

Often, as we expanded our activities, we were challenged by choices we made. In June I went for more training with Steven Rochlitz. Although I had shown I could tolerate the rooms in the Brewster motel, I had had enough of the mold there and chose, instead, to stay at a more modern place not too much further away. When I made a reservation, I was told all rooms except two were taken. One had carpet installed three weeks before. The other had three-year-old carpet that smelled musty because it was on the ground floor. Both options made me nervous. It was the old question of what was more hazardous—mold or chemicals. While I was much improved, this situation involved challenges I did not yet feel comfortable with. I chose the room with the older carpet.

When I arrived at the motel on June fourth, the desk clerk said there was no record of my reservation. The only room available had three-week-old carpet. This news sent me into a panic. I felt uncertain about how I would tolerate two nights in a newly carpeted room. Perhaps I would do fine, but what if I did not? Memories of how exposure to new carpet had precipitated the onset of my environmental illness and all the misery that followed further heightened my anxiety.

I struggled for an hour trying to figure out what to do. When I sat in the room they were offering me, I smelled the carpet, and all the muscles in my body tightened. Unsure what to do, I went out and paced around the motel lobby. I tried calling Patricia to get her input, but there was no answer. The decision was mine alone.

Finally, I decided to try the room with the new carpet. I made it clear to the desk clerk that I had made a reservation, and asked if a room with older carpet became available the next night, could I have it. She said yes and then decided to let me have a room assigned to someone arriving later that night who had made no request about carpet. She would give him mine. Her words sent a wave of relief through me. I gratefully accepted her offer. I would deal with new carpet some time in the future when I felt stronger.

The room I ended up in had minimal carpet odor but smelled of cleaners and mold. Still, it was an improvement over the room I was first offered. I coped by airing the room out and then putting MariEL lines on it. I fell asleep without difficulty. When I woke up the next morning, I had slight muscle aching, which cleared after I did meta-integration exercises. By the second night, I had no symptoms in the room.

The weekend class was the third in a series of workshops on "Touch for Health," a type of energetic healing. The other students included Gloria, a woman with whom I had worked during the first series I attended in November 1991. It was a surprise to see her again. She remembered me as the doctor who had to wear a mask to stay in class and commented on how much healthier and more relaxed I looked than when we first met.

I took my recovery to another level in mid-June when I flew for the first time since becoming sick. My last plane trip had been in 1990 when I went to Hawaii for three weeks. That intense immersion into the high vibrational energy of a week of ocean swims with dolphins, being in the presence of the Avatar known as Ammachi, and two weeks studying qi gong at a Taoist retreat center apparently precipitated the onset of my illness. Having a frequent flier coupon that was about to expire encouraged me to fly again. I was elated to discover I could do so without a problem.

In keeping with what I had learned from my illness, I used the trip to Philadelphia as an opportunity to clear myself of limiting thoughts and beliefs that I held about medicine and healing. As I walked around the University of Pennsylvania, I reminisced on my four years of medical school there and focused on letting go of old beliefs. I then felt a lightening of my energy field and a deeper connection into my body. I honored the importance of letting go of old programming around health and the medical model to make room for new healing methods I was working with and would draw to myself in the future.

Upon returning from Philadelphia, I felt well and shortly thereafter went to an exhibit of transformational artwork. The paintings radiated a tangible vibration that created shifts inside me. By the time I left, I ached all over and had nausea and pain in my belly. Back in Sharon, Patricia, who had not gone to the exhibit, felt nauseous standing next to me. Muscle testing indicated the artwork had produced a clearing. We had adopted an attitude of being thankful for our clearings, but we also questioned how much longer they would go on, how much was there to clear? This experience with the artwork reminded us that there were ways other than the path we had chosen which could stimulate clearings and create healing.

Day-to-day encounters continued to offer opportunities to confront our fears and reprogram our responses to things we had come to view as toxic and dangerous. The office where I worked in Brookline two days a month underwent major renovation, including painting and new carpet. While the adjoining suite was being done first, fumes filtered into my office, bringing on muscle tightness. At the end of the day, I made a point of sitting in the newly redone waiting area to clear my reaction to those chemicals in preparation for when my office was done. I grounded myself, breathed deeply, and gave all the cells of my being permission to release any imbalances I was holding which were associated with my reactions to the chemicals. I then filled the space which had been opened with golden healing energy. By the time I was done, my symptoms were significantly reduced.

Vywamus repeatedly advised Patricia to start doing healing work. He said she would feel better when she did. Although she knew what he said was probably true, she felt neither strong enough nor skilled enough to do so. She chose, instead, to stay in the more familiar setting of private-duty and home-care nursing. She found those jobs boring and restrictive, but their slow pace allowed her to observe how her interactions with others affected her. As she had done with the inner child work, Patricia noted when her energy began to close down and looked at what she had been thinking, what fears and doubts were stimulated, just prior to the experience.

She became aware of behavior patterns which kept her isolated, kept her from really connecting to people and becoming involved with life. For example, she was taken aback when she discovered her illogical reluctance to ask others for help. She judged herself for not being able to handle everything herself.

In the course of her nursing work, Patricia came in contact with substances such as cigarette smoke, new carpet, and perfume, which environmental illness experts said were harmful. She coped by surrounding herself with white light and focusing on being safe in her connection to Spirit. When she did so, she was not bothered by any of these things.

I thought about Michael's December 1991 recommendation that we use daily life as a vehicle for healing. At the time his suggestion seemed too much. It was gratifying to realize we had incorporated this concept and now worked with it on a daily basis.

As Patricia and I traced a path back to health, the news media gave more attention to problems caused by chemicals. There were many stories about the toxic effects of carpets, pesticides, and perfumes. Unusual symptoms reported by people who cleaned up the *Exxon Valdez* Alaskan oil spill and by veterans of the 1991 Gulf War underscored the long-term effects of environmental disasters, and drew more attention to the growing problem of multiple chemical sensitivities.

In a session I had with Sheila on June 28, 1993, Vywamus

talked again about the deep transformation the Earth was undergoing. He said the energies which were stimulating this process had
been referred to by various names, including "Fourth Dimensional
Energy," the "Christ Consciousness," and the "Goddess Energy."
These energies influence everything they touch and aim at creating
deep union of spirit and matter. Whatever is open to this accelera-
tion can move to a higher-vibrational level. Resistance would be
experienced as illness or as a major, perhaps painful, restructuring
of one or more aspects of a person's life.

I asked what role the massive growth in the amount of chemicals used on the planet played in the increased incidence of environmental illness. Vywamus replied that the root cause of any illness is not in the external realm but in the inner experience. He said
what Patricia and I had been learning was that one's internal
process is very deeply connected to the external environment.
Each person is a creator who creates an environment around him-
or herself that reflects the internal process, whatever it may be.

Vywamus gave the example that if people unconsciously see
themselves as victims, they will be drawn to an environment which
creates that experience for them. It is not their external environment
that makes them a victim. It is their internal process which magne-
tizes them to the toxicity. He said you could have two people living
next to a nuclear reactor for years and one develops cancer and the
other does not. All you have to do is look carefully at what they
think, what they feel, how they express themselves, what their
lifestyles are like, and you will find one experiences life as a victim
and the other is very much into saying "yes" to life.

I asked his comments on my recent experience with new carpet
at the motel. Vywamus answered that I had approached myself in a
compassionate way, assessing the situation to see what was right
for me. After I described how intense my fears had been, Vywamus
replied that anyone who is afraid of anything will not be able to run
away from it anymore. They will keep bumping up against it until
they choose no longer to be a victim to it. He added that Mother
Earth had chosen not to be a victim to humanity or to anyone else

in the universe anymore and this was why the global transformation was occurring. In giving up victimization, individuals "own" their own power and state who they are. He noted that Patricia and I were choosing not to be victims anymore; and if we were to move back into a victimization role, it would make us very sick.

We had strong reactions to these latest revelations. Again, we were being told that everything went back to our attitudes and beliefs. Patricia and I had many heated debates about this perspective on how life works. Not yet ready to fully accept Vywamus' view, I asserted that our healing had required interventions on many different energetic levels, including physical, emotional, mental, and spiritual. Patricia also found it hard to take responsibility for everything she experienced but asked where does one draw the line? I agreed, however, that the most profound and lasting changes in our health occurred when we accepted our illness as showing us aspects of ourselves we had denied.

There was truth and simplicity in the notion that recent epidemics of complex, new disorders, like environmental illness and chronic fatigue syndrome, were related to a global tranformational process. The prospect that all of the Earth's people would someday recognize the power of their thoughts to create their reality suggested an astounding, worldwide metamorphosis was possible.

July 1993 marked three years from when I became trapped in environmental illness. I again went to a workshop, this time with Patricia. We spent three-and-a-half days in Maine studying with Vywamus. The channels were Pat Balzer, who had given us a powerful introduction to Vywamus in 1992, and Laura Kramer, who flew in from Oregon. The workshop focused on breaking out of barriers which were erected initially for protection but which now hindered merging with the higher-vibrational energy. Vywamus created many opportunities for our group to experience a magnification of our defense mechanisms and denial so that we could see their effects and choose to let them go, replacing them with attitudes and thoughts which would support continued expansion of our conscious awareness.

New carpet in the meeting room created an unexpected ending to the cycle begun in 1990. My devastating reaction to new rugs then trapped me in environmental illness. Now we both remained symptom-free. As I reviewed the past three years, I felt grateful for what had occurred. My old life had been destroyed, but a new one had begun. Although our evolutionary process would continue at an intense, sometimes painful, almost overpowering pace, now Patricia and I could each move through whatever came up without becoming caught in the amazingly complex prison of environmental illness.

# EPILOGUE

## July 1993—July 1996

"Whatever is wanting to break you and
stop you is your greatest opportunity to
discover a new voice of spirit inside
yourself, because without the adversity
you will not rise."

*The Pleiadian Times*
Summer Solstice 1996

# Epilogue

Freeing ourselves of our chemical sensitivities was a major milestone but certainly not the end of our journey. We came to appreciate our healing as the process of creating a union of Spirit and Matter deep within. Bit by bit we let go of the image of being sick with environmental illness and began to view ourselves as sensitive to the Earth and deeply connected to her and her process. Over the next three years, we broadened our understanding of what we had been through and integrated what we had learned into our daily lives.

Before our introduction to Vywamus in 1992, we had focused extensively on healing our physical bodies and on creating a nontoxic environment for ourselves. We had also begun to touch into energetic aspects of our healing. Then for a year and a half we immersed ourselves in exploring the mind-body-spirit connection. Many forms of energetic healing, including regular bodywork with Adriana, Kristine, and Sheila, as well as personal sessions and classes with Vywamus, channeled by Pat and Sheila, aided us as we moved through the deep clearing process we had chosen to undergo. This comprehensive approach did bring about a healing of our environmental illness. In spite of everything we had done though, Patricia was still plagued by intermittent bouts of fatigue and depression.

In the summer of 1993, we began making periodic trips to Maine to study with Vywamus, channeled by Pat Balzer and Halsey Snow. In this group setting we explored the emotional body at depths we had not before considered possible. In February 1994,

Vywamus began teaching us about connecting to the Goddess energy, the relationship between the Masculine and Feminine, and the cocreative process. Vywamus defined the Feminine energy as the physical and emotional bodies and also as movement, unlimited potential, flow, space, and the unknown. The Masculine was defined as the mental and spiritual bodies, as a focused energy that directs, explores, and *does*. The Feminine simply *is*.

We looked at the many ways that fear and judgment kept us in a separated state and limited the flow of the Feminine. In experiential exercises we were shown repeatedly how beliefs and attitudes we considered to be truths, to be normal, logical, and "the way it is," in fact, cut us off from our own life force and our own potentialities. We would think we had understood, but then would be shown still another way we were saying "NO" to the flow of life, joy, creativity, and potentiality.

Vywamus encouraged us to desire the Feminine and to allow Her full expression of everything She was holding. He said She was holding an enormous amount of pain which She needed to express to the Masculine and to have received by Him. If we could do this, then the Feminine would be able to open up space to draw in the potential we were calling forth.

As we delved deeper into our emotional flows, Patricia's depression intensified. At times it reached such unbearable proportions that we both feared we were making a huge mistake by continuing the spiritual, evolutionary process we had begun. However, Patricia felt compelled to continue, as if she might die if she did not. When we spoke with Vywamus about the scary depths to which she plunged, he replied that many women go through a profound grieving process around the age of forty, as they become aware of a deep emptiness inside themselves. He said this emptiness stems from a lack of true connection to the Masculine, either in themselves, in their partner, or in Spirit. Patricia had turned forty in December 1994.

In February 1995, Patricia spent a few days in Maine without me in an effort to get some help. In a personal session, Pat and

Halsey pointed out to her that most of her difficulties arose from failure to share her internal experiences with me, especially when I said or did things that caused her pain. The problems created by Patricia's unwillingness to give me reflections were twofold. First, I was not given the opportunity to learn how my behavior impacted her; second, the pain and hurt were pushed into her body and manifested days later as physical pain or incapacitation. When this happened, it was almost impossible for us to make a connection between the cause and the effect of the problem.

While Patricia was in Maine, Pat told her she had never before seen a woman so cut off from her own Feminine. Patricia winced at this comment and recalled how she used to view herself as very feminine. She wondered what had happened to her. After returning home, Patricia shared the events of the weekend with me. Gradually, we changed our way of interacting.

For the first four months of 1995, Patricia continued her part-time job as a visiting nurse, but her heart was not in that work. When it became increasingly difficult for her to get out the door in the morning, she decided to quit and leave conventional nursing altogether. By late spring, she was sicker than she had been in years. Her depression was back full force and many other old symptoms returned. Her whole body ached down to her bones. Her head was cloudy. She had no energy. She was nauseated. She had no appetite and no interest in doing anything.

For three days in June, she spent most of her time lying on the futon in the den crying and praying to the Divine Mother for help. She found herself repeatedly saying that she really did want to live, but she did not want to live like this. Nothing I did made much difference. Feeling helpless and at a loss for what to do, I prayed and kept intending to draw to us some way for her to move through the depths of her despair.

On the fourth day, a patient brought me an article on an allergy treatment called the "Nambudripad Allergy Elimination Technique." According to the article, the technique's developer, Dr. Devi S. Nambudripad, considers many illnesses as being caused by allergies. In her view, allergic symptoms occur when energy pathways in the body, known as meridians, are shut down by a particular allergen. Her treatment involves reactivating the affected meridians while the person holds the allergenic substance. She reports results for many people, including individuals with environmental illness and chronic fatigue syndrome.

After discussing the article with Patricia, I decided to attend the next training, which was being held in California ten days later. We were inspired by Dr. Nambudripad's claims, and I was desperate to help Patricia. Since I already was well-versed in the Nambudripad Allergy Elimination Technique's essential elements of Chinese meridian theory and muscle testing, I quickly became comfortable with this method. Testing during the training confirmed my level of recovery. I was strong on nearly all of eighty allergens tested.

Back at home, I tried the technique with Patricia. She tested weak for many items, and responded to the treatments with improvement in her energy level and mood. The biggest gains came after treating her for sugar, B vitamins, and minerals. We also used the technique in our work to examine and change limiting beliefs we held. We found that doing a treatment for a core belief could clear a number of allergies without treating for the specific allergens. The first belief we worked with was "it is not safe to be fully present on the Earth." Patricia kept getting stronger and more energetic with each treatment.

When we spoke with Vywamus about our experiences with this technique, he scolded Patricia for her unwillingness to take responsibility for her struggles with her health. He acknowledged the effectiveness of this method but reminded us the key was not which technique we used. The key, as we had heard before, was in one's choice to be fully present on the Earth. He said she had chosen to fall back into a role of victimization and had left her body for the past few months. Now she had chosen to come back. Period.

Initially, Patricia was greatly angered by what she perceived as Vywamus' lack of compassion. Then she began to explore how she felt victimized by our relationship and by her empathic abilities. As she did so, our relationship changed dramatically. Patricia became progressively more willing to express her thoughts, intuitions, and feelings and to tell me what she sensed in her body. It became clear that often she processed my unconscious thoughts and fears.

At first, I felt attacked by her comments about the pain she experienced in her body and the possible connection to what I was thinking. I was frightened to realize that my thoughts could have such an impact on her, my externalized Feminine. Yet the more I welcomed her expression, the better Patricia felt physically, mentally, and emotionally. By receiving her input, I was able to become aware of a deeper level of unconsciously held, unsupportive thoughts and then to choose different ones, more in alignment with what I wanted in my life.

Patricia and I began to work together offering Nambudripad Allergy Elimination Technique treatments and other energetic work. Thereafter, our healing practice expanded and our financial situation started to move back from the brink of bankruptcy. We were beginning to experience a magical, cocreative partnership, which drew us closer together.

By late 1995, we had grown tired of the process of constantly "looking at our stuff" and chose to have more balance in our healing. Patricia had been putting out intentions daily for many months about what she wanted to experience in our relationship. Each day she invoked love, joy, compassion, gentleness, and other qualities that were continually evolving.

When she spoke with Laura Kramer about a workshop planned for November 1995, Patricia knew we had to go. It turned out to be a small class with only two other participants. Laura channeled Vywamus and a teacher called "Sephron." A key theme was opening our hearts to the compassionate energies of Jesus Sananda. We were both somewhat chagrined as our unconscious resistance to this opening was made public, but we came away from the weekend with a deep sense of peace. Our relationship softened, and we were gentler with one another. We found ourselves shifting from concentrating on inner blocks to focusing with compassion on our wholeness and on manifesting what we wanted in our lives. We began to get clear on what we wanted to create for ourselves.

As we did so, we realized the way we had approached our healing, whether in the form of conventional or alternative medicine or in our spiritual process, had brought us little joy. We both began intending to bring more joy into our lives and soon met Gary Lospaluto, a gentle, compassionate man with a wonderful sense of humor. He had developed a style of inner child work which, in a structured fashion, creates a safe environment where one's inner children can emerge at their own pace and speak if they so choose. During four sessions with Gary, parts of ourselves which had been distorted and shut off came forth and expressed themselves. In allowing this expression and integrating these parts into our conscious awareness, we both contacted new sources of joy and vitality within.

By early 1996 we had synthesized the various modalities we used into a unique approach to help others access their inner resources for healing. We were most gratified by the responses to our work. One woman, who had been severely disabled by chronic fatigue syndrome and environmental illness for six years, experienced a marked increase in her energy level and alleviation of her sensitivities. She reported hearing her son telling a friend he "had his mother back."

Another woman, also with a history of severe chemical sensitivities and chronic fatigue syndrome, had spent most of her days for the previous five years lying on a mat in her living room. She was so weak that she needed to be driven to her appointments and immediately upon entering the office had to lie down. While she benefited greatly from the HEBS exercises (see Glossary) and a series of Nambudripad Allergy Elimination Technique treatments, she made the most progress when we began using the latter method to help her release unconscious, limiting beliefs. Eventually, she was able to identify the beliefs herself and clear them on her own. By April 1996, after seven months of treatment, she was able to drive herself forty-five minutes to our office, had expanded her diet, and could be out of her house for several hours a day.

As our healing work expanded, Patricia developed a greater appreciation for her empathic abilities and her kinesthetic sensitivity. Instead of feeling victimized by her body, she began to honor it as an extraordinary channel. She started using her gifts in our practice, helping people to identify emotional issues they needed to look at.

We also came to appreciate our sensitivities to Mother Earth. For several months in late 1995 and early 1996, Patricia and I repeatedly encountered intense smells of oil. Exhaust fumes entering her rusted out, twelve-year-old car prompted Patricia to retire it. We kept smelling oil in my car, but the mechanic had difficulty finding a source. When he replaced the oil valve covers, however, the odor lessened significantly. The oil smell that we had noticed episodically for four years in our house's forced hot air heating system intensified. While an earlier check of the furnace was negative, in April 1996 leaks were found in the heat exchanger, and the landlord replaced the antiquated unit.

The most striking experience occurred one evening while we were driving home from visiting some friends. The smell of oil on the highway was so strong we were certain there must have been a huge oil spill. The smell lasted for at least ten miles, then suddenly disappeared. What had happened was a mystery to us.

When Patricia questioned Vywamus about the significance of our repeated encounters with petroleum products and their fumes, he replied they were related to a deep clearing process the Earth was undergoing. Because of our sensitivity to the Earth, we sensed what most others would not. He added that by praying for the Earth when we noticed such anomalies, we could help facilitate Her healing. When Patricia asked if this applied to all environmentally sensitive people who had an acute awareness of smells, Vywamus answered with a definite "yes." He suggested that these are people who have the potential to assist in the Earth's healing if they so choose and that they are "trying out for the job."

Later in 1996, Patricia's connection to the Earth again became evident. On June eighth while we were out driving, she suddenly began choking. Patricia asked inside about the cause and felt that there was a serious problem somewhere in China related to the land. She then had a brief image of a nuclear test explosion. Her choking ceased after she prayed for the Earth and for China. The moment we arrived home, our friend Christine, who has strong ties to China, called. She began choking and coughing as soon as Patricia picked up the phone. Patricia told Christine to pray for China; and when she did so, her choking stopped. The next day newspapers reported that China had detonated an underground nuclear weapon in the 20-to-80-kiloton range at Lop Nor in north-western Xinjiang province.

In December 1995 we had begun focusing our energies on completing this book. We worked intensely at all hours of the day or night and had no time for cooking. As a result, we ate nothing but restaurant and take-out food—pizza, Chinese, Indian, Thai—whatever we found that was easy and sounded good. We wrote whenever we could and frequently were up until three o'clock, drinking coffee and eating chocolate at midnight. We had no fixed schedule and did no yoga or meditation. We often felt conflicted about letting go of the many rules about what to eat or do until we realized that we felt good and had lots of energy.

After four months of eating that way, Patricia and I began wanting nothing but macrobiotic food. With no time to cook, we were grateful for pre-made macrobiotic meals available at the health food store and a great macrobiotic restaurant in Cambridge. It was a very different experience to eat this food because it was what we wanted rather than because we thought it was what we had to eat to get well. We had achieved a state of being able to allow our desires to determine our course of action regardless of the dogma "out there" about what one should do to stay healthy and spiritually connected.

Vywamus' and Michael's insistence that we create our reality with our thoughts, that our judgments keep us in a separated state, that it is our choice to remain in that separated state, and that we are the only ones stopping our flow, now made sense. We had become living proof of these teachings which years before had made us so angry. It became clear, too, that as we allowed our life force to flow in the cocreative process, self-imposed limitations fell away. Writing this book had become our "spiritual practice," and the practice was really about connecting to ourselves and one another, and doing what we WANTED to do, doing what brought us joy, and expressing ourselves freely and fully.

For some time we had known we wanted to move when the Sharon lease ended on July first. In the midst of finishing this book we began house hunting, again. We made another list of what we wanted in a house. This time we concentrated more on how the house would feel and how it would support us rather than on whether it had specific features which we viewed as safe and nontoxic. We used our intentions to find a place where we would enjoy living, which would nourish and support us as we expanded our lives, a place which would feel like home.

Although people said we would have difficulty finding a house rental in the area where we were looking in southern New Hampshire, we chose to hold our focus on what we wanted to manifest and were shown six possibilities in one day. We were very pleased with the house we chose, a spacious contemporary with a fluid flow of energy and a feeling of home. The fact that it had wall-to-wall carpet throughout both frightened and intrigued me.

During all of June we worked feverishly, alternating between completing this book and packing. We realized that in order to conclude this latest part of our healing we had to leave Sharon, where our most intense inner work had been done; but, in order to leave Sharon, we had to finish this book. We worried about how we would ever accomplish all there was to be done and were grateful when unexpected help arrived.

Living in Sharon, surrounded by the Audubon Sanctuary, had allowed us to cultivate our relationship with the animal kingdom. Over the course of four years we came to appreciate the animals' ability to give us information through the reflective process, if we were willing to receive it. Talking to the animals, as many people do, usually did not bring us the insights we sought. When a particular animal showed up repeatedly, or in an unusual manner, we referred to the cards in *Medicine Cards* by Jamie Sams and David Carson to understand the message they brought us. We thus received help from coyote, fox, deer, snake, crow, spider, hawk, and many others. While in Sharon, we had made a conscious choice not to intentionally kill any living creature, and we found that flies, mosquitoes, and even wasps that wandered into the house would allow us to catch them in a jar and put them outside.

The unexpected help I referred to arrived in May, when hundreds of tiny ants invaded our kitchen. They showed up in droves on the counters, covering one portion at a time and working their way around the room in a clockwise fashion. They appeared in one section for several days and then moved to the area to the right.

To cope with the ants, Patricia first tried speaking with them and their devas, or nature spirits. Then she drew energetic lines and asked the ants to respect our space and not cross the lines. Each time the ants lessened in number but only briefly. After she had me talk to the ants and draw lines, there again was only a temporary reprieve. Each morning Patricia tried to create some usable space on the counters by gently brushing the ants into a jar, putting them outside, and asking them not to return. Regardless of our best efforts, the invasion continued unabated; I resorted to ant traps, but to no avail. Patricia soon threw the traps out, insisting there must be a better way. However, even she was reaching her limit.

A conversation Patricia had with Sheila Simon two days later gave us another avenue to pursue. When Sheila mentioned Vywamus' recent comments about ants being particularly telepathic, Patricia suspected the ants might be trying to communicate something. The following morning she went to their latest location, on the stove, and stated her desire to receive whatever they had to tell her. As Patricia tuned in to the ants, she felt enveloped by a very strong, pleasant energy for about thirty seconds. She sought a way to interpret this information, but no words came to her. She then thanked the ants, gathered them up, and put them outside. The next day she was able to write a portion of this book on which she had been stuck for two weeks.

Patricia recognized the connection between the energy from the ants and a freeing up of her writing the next morning, when the ants again were on the stove and she repeated her communication with them. Before she put the ants outside, she asked me to connect to them as well. Then for the first time in weeks, the ants stopped coming. Several days later when our writing was again blocked, the ants reappeared. When we asked for whatever the ants had to give us, we felt another surge of energy, a piece for the book came, and then the ants were gone. This process took place four more times. We completed the manuscript and sent it to Barbara Clow of Bear & Company on June twenty-eighth. Thereafter, the tiny ants stopped coming.

Two days later, as if to make sure we knew it was time to leave, a column of big ants appeared, marched single-file up the wall, and repeatedly circled the kitchen clock. When we asked if they had anything to bring us, their transmission of energy gave us a much needed boost to complete our packing. How simple. No pesticides, no poisons. Just communication, connection, and receiving what they had to offer.

Our move to New Hampshire went well despite concerns about the wall-to-wall carpet and a couple other features of the new house. I have enjoyed returning to the state where I grew up. Leaving Sharon and settling into our new home has been a perfect time to reflect on what we learned over the last six years.

When I joined with Patricia in 1990 to overcome environmental illness, I had no conscious awareness of the complexity of the journey we were embarking upon. Perhaps at a soul level, however, I always knew. Patricia reminded me that after we first met it took me three weeks to call her. We speculated that at some level I was considering whether I wanted to go through all the pain and agony which lay ahead. But the journey which led me into the extremely compressed state of being trapped in environmental illness ultimately led to freedom from constraints I had unknowingly placed on myself.

All of my study of medicine and psychiatry, of Eastern philosophies and spiritual practices, as well as of many healing arts did not give me the tools I needed to heal this illness. Patricia's nursing education and years of practice were of little help in the recovery process. To get well we had to venture far outside our comfort zones and let go of all of our notions about illness and health. We did not know that we did not know how to feel our feelings. We thought we were feeling them. We did not realize the degree to which we were disconnected from ourselves and our surroundings, or that this lack of connection was killing us.

Healing our physical bodies with such interventions as special diets, herbs, and a toxin-free environment was an important first step in our recovery; but until we understood what we were trying to show ourselves, we remained locked in a state of victimization and fear, unable to return to a full and productive life. The many avenues we pursued in our healing allowed us to slowly release layer after layer of physical and emotional toxicity and to become aware of the bigger picture of our environmental illness. Looking at the body as a metaphor that reflects our thoughts and beliefs back to us, we are impressed by the simplicity of the message we were sending ourselves: It does not feel safe to be present in the fullness of who we are here, on the Earth, in a physical body.

Humanity has made a choice to evolve beyond the separated state in which we currently find ourselves. To do so requires the Divine Feminine, the Mother, the Goddess in ourselves and all around us. The mass consciousness of the Feminine holds the experience of being contaminated, poisoned, and abused by the disconnected male and feels victimized by this experience. Environmental illness can be viewed as the physical manifestation, on an individual level, of this aspect of the Feminine, which needs healing.

Environmental illness gave Patricia and me the opportunity to feel on a personal, visceral level how we all are connected to each other and to our surroundings. The degree to which humanmade toxins pervade our environment became terrifyingly clear. But chemicals, poisons, and nuclear waste are not at the heart of the problem, and eliminating them is not the full solution. They are a reflection of the Masculine's attempt to control his physical environment, the Feminine, while in a state of separation.

The various substances that have appeared as part of efforts to bring "convenience" to modern life will not disappear from our reality until enough people understand at the core of their being the deleterious effects they are having on our world. If Vywamus' prediction comes true, that over the next twenty-five years nearly everyone on the Earth will have some form of environmental illness, humanity will have the motivation to find new ways of getting our needs met without destroying the environment.

Since Patricia and I became ill, there has been a significant increase in the incidence of environmental illness and chronic fatigue syndrome. Already a variety of less toxic, alternative products are being made available in response to the needs of chemically sensitive individuals and the preference of those who want to use environmentally friendly products. Heretofore unknown solutions to the many, apparently insolvable, problems facing humanity will become available as people touch more deeply into the unknown Feminine energy which is flooding the Earth with increasing intensity. This same energy influx is also stimulating evolution of each individual's psychospiritual nervous system. This process can manifest in what may be interpreted as diseases of the nervous system, which is closely tied to the immune system. Vywamus has suggested that we shall see many new and unusual nervous system disorders, particularly in women, as the planetary transformation continues.

As Patricia and I move back to mainstream life, we are continuously challenged to reevaluate our beliefs about what is safe, what is healthy, what will harm us, what are environmentally responsible or irresponsible actions, and how can we live in modern society and still respect the sacredness of all life and the delicate balance of this beautiful planet. We have returned to a more "normal" lifestyle.

Patricia again uses makeup and has her hair colored. We are able to wear new clothes, go shopping, eat in restaurants, and travel. We even have fun once in a while!

We are thankful to be strong enough now to make choices about interacting with our environment not out of fear of being poisoned but out of respect for all living creatures and from an understanding of the impact of our actions. Environmental illness was for both of us a vehicle which awakened us to our disconnected state and stimulated a desire for connection to ourselves and the Feminine, and for a global healing that we had not previously thought of seeking. We are grateful for all we have experienced and offer our story to assist others in their return to the WHOLENESS.

*"Every part of the Earth is sacred to my people. We are part of the Earth and it is part of us. We know the white people do not understand our ways. One portion of land is the same to them as the next, for they are strangers who come in the night and take from the land whatever they need. This we know. The Earth does not belong to humans; humans belong to the Earth. All things are connected like the blood which unites one family. Whatever befalls the Earth befalls the children of the Earth. Humans do not weave the web of life; they are merely a strand in it. Whatever they do to the web, they do to themselves."*

Chief Seattle, 1854

From a speech given in his native Duwamish tongue to his tribal assembly in the Pacific Northwest in response to an offer by the United States government to buy his people's land. Adapted from "Environmental Illness: A Special Report" by Richard Leviton in *Yoga Journal*, November/ December 1990.

# Appendix I

*Limbic Dysregulation, an Etiological Theory for Chronic Fatigue Syndrome and Environmental Illness, and its Relationship to the Evolutionary Process*

When cases of people suffering with what is now called chronic fatigue syndrome appeared in the 1980s, the response of the medical establishment was generally to say either it did not exist or it must be psychological. As more people developed this disorder and research continued, by 1994 there was consensus that chronic fatigue syndrome existed, but its cause remained undetermined.[1] Environmental illness has had a similar history, just a few years later in coming. Again, with symptoms involving multiple systems of the body, including the brain, and many subjective complaints, there has been a tendency for physicians and researchers to say either there is no problem or it is all in the mind of the patient. In our experiences in our own healing process and those of a number of clients, we view environmental illness and chronic fatigue syndrome as holistic illnesses that call for a broader understanding of the relationship between mind, body, emotions, and spirit. This appendix discusses limbic dysregulation, one etiological theory which offers the possibility of a broader understanding of how these disorders are created.

Jay A. Goldstein, M.D., director of the Chronic Fatigue Syndrome Institutes in Anaheim and Santa Monica, California, views multiple chemical sensitivity syndrome and chronic fatigue syndrome as "two related expressions of a central limbic regulatory dysfunction."[2] The limbic system is a complex neural network. Its major structures include the hippocampus and amygdala, both located in the medial part of the anterior temporal lobe of the brain. In his book, *Chronic Fatigue Syndromes:*

*The Limbic Hypothesis,* Dr. Goldstein reviews the anatomy and physiology of the limbic system. Of note is its role as a "buffer between the internal and external world." It sends projections both to specialized areas of the cerebral cortex which are involved with integration of the autonomic nervous system and to instinctual parts of the nervous system in the lower brain stem, spinal cord, and autonomic nervous system.[3] Dr. Goldstein proposes that through these connections the limbic system acts as a neuroregulator for the body.[4]

One difficulty in the diagnosis of both chronic fatigue syndrome and environmental illness is that they often involve numerous, seemingly unrelated, symptoms. In Dr. Goldstein's view, most of their symptoms can be explained by limbic system dysfunction.[5] Areas with which the limbic system is involved include memory, emotions, sleep, stress responses, and regulation of endocrine and immune functions.

Drawing on the multiple chemical sensitivity syndrome literature and on research in neurotoxicology, occupational medicine, and biological psychiatry, Iris Bell, M.D., and her colleagues have proposed a model of multiple chemical sensitivity syndrome (MCS) based on kindling of the olfactory and limbic systems. "Kindling" refers to the ability of a repeated, intermittent stimulus that initially does not elicit a response, eventually to induce a motor seizure from application of the same stimulus. The olfactory pathways and certain limbic structures are especially vulnerable to kindling, which may be chemical or electrical.[6] Studies in monkeys have shown that injection of an organophosphate pesticide at a lower dose (1 μg/kg) weekly for ten weeks had the same effect on the EEG one year later as did one larger dose (5μg/kg) of the same substance.[7] Lack of a blood-brain barrier in the olfactory system provides a means by which chemicals can gain direct access to the olfactory bulb and other parts of the central nervous system via the nasal mucosa.

Bell et al. use kindling to refer, in nonepileptic humans, to "permanent increases in limbic neuronal excitability and associated behaviors via repeated subthreshold stimulation."[8] This description is consistent with the experiences of many people who develop MCS following chronic low-level exposure to chemicals. They may have repeated exposure to a substance without obvious effects, but then one more exposure results in a marked and persistent heightened reactivity which may expand to include sensitivity to other chemicals as well.

Robert Post, M.D.,[9] first discussed kindling in relation to affective disorders. He proposed it as a mechanism in early episodes of affective disorders by which psychosocial stressors created changes in the brain leading to increased likelihood of later episodes occurring independent of external stressors. While Bell et al. acknowledge the role of psychosocial stressors in kindling, their article focuses on the role various environmental chemicals such as pesticides, flame retardants, formaldehyde, acetone, benzene, and ozone can play in inducing kindling in limbic structures. These trigger and/or perpetuate affective and cognitive disorders as well as related somatic disorders to give the presentation seen in MCS. They suggest that those most vulnerable to kindling from low-level environmental chemicals would be those genetically predisposed to certain affective spectrum disorders such as depression. Within this model, psychiatricly healthy individuals could also develop chemically induced symptoms, but only from higher concentrations or longer exposure periods.[10]

The work of Goldstein and Bell et al. suggests that to understand and treat environmental illness and chronic fatigue syndrome, it is essential to take a broad view of these disorders, which will incorporate physical, mental, and emotional factors. Based on our experiences with these disorders we recommend some additional considerations. First, as the Earth passes through what has been referred to as a time of clearing at a planetary level, individuals will be stimulated to release traumatic memories from their present and past lives, a clearing of the karmic bank so to speak. The experience of these memories may stimulate the limbic system and heighten sensitivities. Second, as the higher-vibrational energies that began increasing in the 1980s continue to accelerate, they may also increase limbic arousal and thereby increase sensitivities. We have repeatedly had individuals, independently of each other, complain of increased symptoms at times when various sources have indicated that major energy influxes were occurring. Third, the limbic system is intimately involved with the glandular system of the body in general and particularly with the pituitary gland and the pineal gland, which have been identified as being connected to the chakra system. Various teachers have talked about a new twelve-chakra system being layered in. It seems possible that as the new chakras are layered in, that process could stimulate the limbic system, leading to a heightening of sensitivities or contributing to the process of kindling.

[1] Anthony Komaroff, M.D., speaking at the annual meeting of the Massachusetts CFIDS Association on June 5, 1994.

[2] J.A. Goldstein, "Ask the Doctor," *CFIDS Chronicle*, Winter 1994, p.49.

[3] J.A. Goldstein, *Chronic Fatigue Syndromes:The Limbic Hypothesis* (Binghamton, NY: The Haworth Press, 1993), pp.24-27.

[4] Ibid., p.36.

[5] Ibid., p.39-87.

[6] I.R. Bell et al., "An Olfactory-Limbic Model of Multiple Chemical Sensitivity Syndrome: Possible Relationships to Kindling and Affective Spectrum Disorders," *Biological Psychiatry* 32 (1992), pp.218-242.
Ibid., p.220.

[7] J.L. Burchfiel and F.H. Duffy, "Organophosphate neurotoxicity: Chronic effects of sarin on the electroencephalogram of monkeys and man," *Neurobehavioral Toxicol Teratol* 4 (1982), pp.767-778.

[8] Bell et al., op. cit., p.221.

[9] R.M. Post, "Minireview. Intermittent versus continuous stimulation: Effect of time interval on the development of sensitization or tolerance." *Life Sci* 26 (1980), pp.1275-1282.

[10] Bell et al., op. cit., p.222.

# Appendix II

## *An Introduction to Kinesiology*

Kinesiology, or muscle testing, is a method to assess the status of the human energy field through changes in muscle strength. One generally used form of muscle testing involves having a tester press down on the arm of a testee while an item is placed next to the testee's body. If the testee's arm goes weak, the item is weakening for the subject and should be avoided. Muscle testing can also be used in energy balancing to bring the body into greater balance. This section of the appendix aims at giving some background on kinesiology and providing you with information so that you can begin experimenting with it if you so choose.

Kinesiology is based on the increasingly recognized fact that humans have not only a physical body but also an energy field, radiating out anywhere from inches to feet, which is the sum of the interactions of the various bodies—mental, emotional, physical, spiritual, and others—of which they are made. As various tangible factors, such as a food, or less tangible factors, such as a thought or an emotion, are brought within a person's energy field, this person's energy is either strengthened or weakened. This change affects the electrical system, which impacts the nervous system, and then can be measured by whether an indicator muscle tests strong or weak. A similar principle of measuring subtle changes in the electrical system of the body to gain information about functioning is used in both lie detectors and biofeedback devices.

Much of kinesiology as it is known today grows out of the work of George Goodheart, D.C., in the 1960s. One of his most significant findings was an energetic association between specific muscles and the meridians of acupuncture theory. There are twelve meridians, each of

229

which is associated with an organ of the body—the lungs, large intestine, stomach, spleen, heart, small intestine, bladder, kidney, pericardium, triple warmer, gall bladder, and liver. Recognition of the muscle/meridian/ organ connection gives healers a means to assess the functioning of the meridian/organ systems and to energetically balance them.

Dr. Goodheart's work became known as "applied kinesiology," the study of which has been limited to professionals. John Thie, D.C., a colleague of Dr. Goodheart, adapted the findings of applied kinesiology for use by lay people and published his book, *Touch for Health,* in 1973. The book's aim was to bring the benefits of muscle testing and energy balancing to the general population. Dr. Thie has had significant success in that regard, with over two million copies sold in more than forty-two countries worldwide. In the 1980s and 1990s, many different forms of kinesiology have emerged from Dr. Thie's findings, as people from many walks of life have learned muscle testing and applied it to their particular areas of interest including health care, psychotherapy, nutrition, music, and sports psychology.[1]

Starting in chapter 8, we mentioned muscle testing frequently in our book. Our experiences with physicist and kinesiologist Steven Rochlitz were a turning point in our recovery. He used kinesiology to identify whether such factors as parasites, bacteria, viruses, and Candida were adversely affecting us, and to find what would be safe and effective to help us eliminate them and to balance us energetically. After our sessions with Steven and my taking his training, we consistently used kinesiology to determine which foods, supplements, herbs, and other substances were beneficial for us and which were not.

Muscle testing is as much an art as a science. It is a skill developed with practice which allows us to tune into energy changes in others and in themselves. Muscle testing can be done either with another individual or for one's self (self-testing). The focus here is on testing with another individual, using the anterior deltoid muscle of the arm as the indicator muscle; many of the same principles also apply to self-testing.

Guidelines for testing:

1. Tester (**A**) and testee (**B**) should be relaxed and open to any result.
2. **A** and **B** should stand erect and not use any muscles in addition to the one that is being focused on in the testing.
3. Keep breathing throughout the testing.

4. Both individuals should be looking straight ahead and not engage one another in eye contact.

5. Prior to testing it can be helpful to balance your energy to increase the body's awareness of the process by touching certain acupuncture points as follows:

a. one hand touches the navel and the thumb and two fingers of the other hand rub the points below the collarbone-breastbone junction on both sides.

b. one hand touches the navel and the other rubs points above and below the upper and lower lips.

c. one hand touches the navel and the other rubs the tailbone.

Together these three are known as "switching corrections."

6. If **B** has any problem with the left arm, do not use it.

7. If any pain develops, stop at that point.

8. Do not test if **B** is hungry or thirsty.

9. Relax and enjoy the process which is one of discovery and healing.

In the testing procedure itself, **A** stands to the side of **B**, whose left arm is held straight in front of the body at a forty-five degree angle from the floor. **A** rests his or her left hand lightly on **B**'s right shoulder for balance and places two fingers of his or her right hand on **B**'s left forearm just above the wrist. The testing procedure is not a contest of strength but an effort to acquire information. It has been said that muscle testing is 80% mental and 20% physical.

It is helpful for **A** to do some initial testing to gauge **B**'s response. Each time just before applying pressure to **B**'s arm, **A** says "hold." Then **A** applies a pressure of ten to fifteen pounds for no more than two seconds or a distance of two inches. The pressure is applied slowly, peaking at the end of two seconds. **B** tries to oppose the pressure and keep his or her arm up. The aim is to see how **B**'s arm responds to that amount of pressure. Should the arm weaken, it is not necessary to push it very far beyond the point where it goes weak.

Some initial calibration can be done by having **B** say "yes" and testing, and then say "no" and testing. The arm should remain strong in response to "yes" and go weak in response to "no." If the results are opposite to this, **B** may need more switching correction as described above or perhaps the overenergy correction described below. **A** can further gauge **B**'s response by having the person say "my name is (his or her name)."

The response should be strong. And then when **B** says "my name is (not his or her name)," the response should be weak.

Before proceeding further, it is also helpful to test after having **B** say "I want to be well" and "I want to be sick." If **B** tests strong to the former statement and weak to the latter statement, proceed with the testing. If **B** tests weak to the former and strong to the latter, an imbalance, which Steven Rochlitz refers to as "overenergy," is present and a correction should be done. Rochlitz likens this reverse response to the person who has worked for twenty-four hours straight and then, when given the chance to sleep, is unable to do so because he or she is too overtired to sleep.[2]

He describes the correction as follows:

1. Cross the legs at the ankle (left over right).
2. Put the arms straight out with the hands back to back.
3. Lift the right hand over the left so that the palms are facing each other.
4. Clasp the fingers and fold the hands and arms in and rest them on your chest.
5. As you breathe in, touch the tongue behind the upper teeth; as you breathe out, touch the tongue behind the lower teeth. As you do so, picture yourself being healthy and well.
6. Do this for one to two minutes and then redo the overenergy test.

"Being well" should now test strong and "being sick" should now test weak. About 5% of the population will not test strong at this point; and they need to place their hands and feet in the position opposite to that described above.[3]

I have found the overenergy correction to be extremely helpful in assisting people to begin to gain more benefit from their efforts to get well.

The overenergy correction can be applied not only to the general case given above but also to specific situations. For example, someone could be tested for the statement, "I want to be free of my allergies," and then for the statement, "I want my allergies to stay the same." Testing weak for the first statement and strong for the second statement would indicate the person had a specific overenergy imbalance regarding being free of allergies. The correction is the same as described above, but in this case the person focuses on being free of allergies, or any other issue being worked on, for a minute or two. Correcting the overenergy imbalance is not necessarily going to eliminate the person's allergies, but it will allow the person's energies to be more fully aligned with his or her efforts to be allergy free.

Having done the above preliminaries, **A** can proceed with the testing for specific items, such as a food, by holding it next to **B**'s body and muscle testing. Various authorities recommend different locations to place the test substance. Some have the testee put it in his or her mouth. The people we work with tend to be quite sensitive so we follow the method of Steven Rochlitz, who recommends holding the test item in the testee's energy field an inch or two away from the body. He describes six different main test areas including next to the liver and next to the spleen.[4] If the arm goes weak, it indicates that the food is weakening for that person and it should be avoided. Similarly, testing can be done for other items such as fabrics, or lotions, or anything else **B** might come in contact with. If one or more items test weak, **B** may want to reverse the situation through an energetic treatment.

Testing can also focus on asking questions. In that case a question is asked of the body and the arm is tested. The precise wording of the question is critical. Testing can be done to ask which among various options would be most helpful for the person's health at a particular time. Or, if a reaction is occurring, testing can be used to ask its origin. In the case of asking questions, a question is asked and immediately the arm is tested. When asking questions, "yes" is indicated by **B**'s left arm becoming weak and going down. "No" is indicated by the arm staying strong and staying up. This is different from testing by placing items next to the body. A key point in testing by asking questions is to phrase the question so that it has a yes or no answer.

Patricia and I found testing by asking questions helpful in many situations, but it was especially helpful when we were having acute symptoms and we were trying to find out the causes. Were the symptoms part of a reaction? If so, what were we reacting to? Was it emotional or related to an influx of energy? Should we leave the environment we were in to escape a toxin? Eventually, in our healing, the answers indicated that the symptoms we were having which had previously been part of a reaction were now a clearing that was part of our becoming well. We approched whatever answers we received with openmindedness, at times facilitated by doing the overenergy correction, and also with compassion for ourselves. We viewed the results from muscle testing as information we added to our data base from which to decide what we wanted to do.

The material presented here is a brief introduction to the vast and rapidly expanding area of kinesiology. You are encouraged to experiment with it as a means to accessing your own inner wisdom. As part of the process the Earth and humanity are moving through, people will eventually have ongoing, direct access to that information and such tools as muscle testing will not be needed. For now, kinesiology is one way to deepen that knowing.

[1] B. Dewe and J. Dewe, *Professional Health Provider I: Advanced Specialized Kinesiology Methods* (Auckland, New Zealand: Professional Health Practice Workshops, 1990), pp. x-xi.

[2] S. Rochlitz, *Allergies and Candida with the Physicist's Rapid Solution* (Mahopac, NY: Human Ecology Balancing Sciences, Inc., 1991), pp. 219-220.

[3] Reprinted by permission of Human Ecology Balancing Sciences, Inc., P.O. Box 737, Mahopac, NY 10541, (914) 228-4162, publishers of *Allergies and Candida with the Physicist's Rapid Solution*.

[4] Rochlitz, ibid., pp. 113-115.

# Appendix III

## *Techniques for Energetic Self-Care*

As described in parts II and III of this book, we found a variety of energetic self-care techniques helpful in our recovery process. We are currently completing a workbook which will give a more comprehensive presentation of the tools we used. We include those described below for your enjoyment and benefit.

### GROUNDING
First and foremost, find ways to enjoy being in your body and to ground your energy.

Stand with bare feet on the ground.

Lie on the ground.

Walk in nature.

Swim, or sit in a whirlpool.

Have bodywork or a massage.

Dance.

Perform exercise that you enjoy—we are not talking about riding an exercise bicycle while watching television.

Yoga.

Tai Chi.

Massage your feet.

### TONING AND/OR CHANTING
Sound can have a profound healing effect on the body. Many spiritual traditions include chanting as part of their practice, as a way to bring about a trance state, or to connect to the Divine prior to meditation. Shamans in all cultures use sound in their healing rituals.

Toning is simply allowing your self to make sounds—whatever sounds want to come out. They can be quiet, soft, almost internal sounds, moderately loud sounds, or whoops, hollers, and yahoos. You might laugh, or cry, or yell and scream. Higher-pitched sounds affect the higher chakras, while lower-pitched sounds affect the lower ones. If you sit still while making sounds, you can begin to feel that different tones and pitches affect different parts of the body.

People are often shy about making spontaneous sounds, especially when they have been ill and isolated, or if they grew up in an oppressive atmosphere where it was not okay to make noise. If your living situation is one where you feel you would be imposing on others by making such sounds, your car can be a great place to be alone and tone. Toning can really shift your energy! Give it a try!

## GOLDEN EGG MEDITATION

This is a meditation Vywamus suggested for Patricia to help her start creating energetic boundaries for herself:

See yourself surrounded by an egg of golden light that extends out about twelve inches from your body in all directions. Focus on that light until you are really aware of it. You see it, feel it, or just know it is there. This is your aura. Bring blue-green light in through the top of the egg and let it fill the space all around you. See the light cleansing the space between you and the outermost part of the egg. Now imagine a little door in the front of the egg in the area of your belly. The door opens and allows the light and the transmuted energy to leave the egg, and yet does not allow anything to come in. Repeat this several times until you experience a sense of peace and relaxation. Now fill the egg one last time with whatever color comes to mind. Surround yourself again with the golden egg. Slowly open your eyes. Be aware of the golden egg surrounding you throughout the day.

Doing this meditation on a regular basis can help you set up your energetic boundaries and remind you that you need not interact with and process another person's energy unless you choose to do so.

## CORD CUTTING

Mary Elizabeth Jochmans has written several books including one we have used extensively called *Changing Cords of Fear into Chords of Love*. In it she discusses her views on how people get energetically intertwined with one another in a codependent manner that does not support either person in their evolutionary process. (A similar concept is written about in James Redfield's popular book, *The Celestine Prophecy*.) With Mary's permission, we offer her basic cord-cutting technique. We have found the meditations in her book to be powerful, effective, and compassionate methods to allow people to feel their own energies, to establish energetic boundaries, and to create relationships which are supportive for themselves at the same time being supportive of others. [Note:"cord" here refers to an energetic connection.]

## BASIC CORD CUTTING[1]

The following guided imagery is one that may be used to release any cords—physical, mental, emotional, spiritual, psychic, astral, karmic, or etheric—that you choose to release.

Remember to follow each step and do each part. It is important to learn the lesson you chose to learn; you could draw another situation just like it into our life and repeat the same situation, possibly more intensely.

## CORD-CUTTING GUIDED IMAGERY

1. Get into a relaxed position either sitting or lying down. See, feel, become aware on all levels of the person (place, thing, or situation) you wish to release cords from. See it in front of you in all its detail. Image it as clearly as possible in your mind's eye. If you do not "see" anything try feeling it. Sense it. Smell it. Make it as real as possible.

2. Gradually become aware of the energy connections between you. See these as cords, threads, or webs and lines of energy running from the other person (place, thing, or situation) connecting to different parts of your body. Become aware also of all the cords, threads, and webs going from you to the other person (place, thing, or situation). Look to see if there are cords attached to your ankles, feet, or knees. Look for cords attached to your shoulders, neck, or back. Be sure to look behind you for cords. Look for cords attached to your head, heart, throat, solar plexus (stomach), sexual, and root (base of spine) centers. All these cords represent attachments and expectations. Some or all of these may be present. They may be thick or thin. Light or heavy. Dark or light.

3. After becoming aware of all energy cords between you and the other person (place, thing, or situation) in your mind's eye, see a sword of crystal blue-white light appear in your right hand. With this sword, gen-

tly and lovingly cut all the cords—physical, emotional, mental, spiritual, psychic, astral, etheric, and karmic—running between you and the other person (place, thing, or situation) and from this person to you. Don't forget the cords behind you. If a cord seems too big or hard to cut with a sword, you may want to use an axe, saw, or hatchet instead.

4. After cutting all the cords, see the sword or other tool disappear. Now in your left hand see a burning torch of crystal blue-white light. With it cauterize (burn) all the ends of the cords you have cut so they cannot be reattached.

5. As the torch and cords disappear ask that all the empty spaces left behind where the cords had been attached be filled with Golden Energy and Love, both in you and in the other person. Feel the empty spaces within you filling with warmth and light and energy.

6. Now ask that all the seals for all the energy bodies—physical, emotional, mental, spiritual, astral, karmic, and etheric—be brought into place and the energy bodies be brought into balance, wholeness, and communication with each other. Relax and feel the sense of release, relief, safeness, and wholeness. Breathe deeply. Relax.

7. And now ask that you be shown what lessons it is you chose to learn by drawing this person (place, thing, or situation) into your life.

8. Give yourself time to receive this information. Close by saying, "It is good, it is done, so let it be. So it is. Peace" or some other words of your own choosing.

9. Be sure to thank yourself and Spirit for this good work. (Those who are very used to depending on cords for their functioning may initially feel very alone. Be sure to use all the Golden Energy and Love from Spirit to fill up any space that feels empty inside.)

HUMAN ECOLOGY BALANCING SCIENCES (HEBS) MAESTRO[2]

The book *Allergies and Candida with the Physicist's Rapid Solution* has several chapters on self-help exercises which are particularly helpful for people with allergies, candida, chemical sensitivities, and chronic fatigue syndrome. We reprint here one that benefits the heart by integrating and strengthening it. The exercise is called the HEBS Maestro and involves a movement that musical conductors (who in many cases live to old age) do regularly.

1. With the elbows high and out to the side a bit, trace (with your hands, not your eyes) two "C's" that are back to back.

2. Hum a note or a tune.

3. After thirty seconds, slowly, visually track (look at) all the points along a large circle in front of you, as you continue the exercise. First gaze along a clockwise direction and then counterclockwise.[3]

This exercise can be done at your own pace, following the directions as well as you can. Rochlitz reports that benefits associated with doing this exercise and another heart integration exercise in his book have included normalizing of blood pressure and improved circulation. He cautions, however, that if the blood pressure imbalance is related to diet that factor must be addressed as well.[4]

---

[1] Reprinted, with minor adaptations, by permission of Mary Elizabeth Jochmans, Alma Tara Publishing, P.O. Box 4230, Blaine, WA 98231-4230, (360) 371-3134, from *Changing Cords of Fear into Chords of Love*.

[2] Reprinted by permission of Human Ecology Balancing Sciences, Inc., P.O. Box 737, Mahopac, NY 10541, (914) 228-4162, from *Allergies and Candida with the Physicist's Rapid Solution* by Steven Rochlitz.

[3] S. Rochlitz, op. cit., p. 139.

[4] Ibid., pp. 140-141.

# Appendix IV

*Thirteen Observations on Healing Environmental Illness and Chronic Fatigue Syndrome*

• Each person has his or her own unique healing process. Not everyone has to go through all we went through. Various people have healed environmental illness and chronic fatigue syndrome through strictly physical means, such as nutritional and environmental changes, or by treating a parasite infection, a Candida overgrowth, and/or other gastrointestinal imbalances.

• It is our observation that the nervous systems of these indiviuals can be profoundly affected, be it from chemical toxicity, emotional stress, the onset of a transformative spiritual evolutionary process, or some combination of these factors. We recommend that evaluation and treatment of these clients be as noninvasive as possible, and that the early focus be on balancing and supporting the nervous system. We feel that substances should be introduced into the bodies of such clients with great caution. Medications, supplements, herbs, homeopathic remedies, intradermal allergy testing, and EPD all have the potential to overload this type of individual. For both of us, several rounds of intradermal allergy testing were followed by significant increases in our sensitivities. Several of our clients described similar experiences. The Limbic Dysregulation Hypothesis described in Appendix I provides a rationale for why intradermal testing done intermittently could produce a heightening of sensitivities. Although we are not aware of any research on this topic, we recommend considering other less invasive, more balancing processes before employing such techniques. Patients may then better tolerate these more aggressive processes better, or perhaps find them unnecessary.

• Patients with environmental illness and chronic fatigue syndrome also frequently are found to have imbalances of one or more neurotransmitters or hormones. We have read various articles speculating on the effects of the many chemicals in our food and environment on these systems. Pregnant women often experience a heightened sensitivity to smell, and  pregnancy is another life experience that has been noted to precede these disorders. We also note that various writings about people experiencing an intense process of spiritual enlightenment such as the rising of kundalini energies or shamanistic rites of passage describe that these people become extremely sensitive. We would again like to note that many spiritual practices and ancient healing techniques can bring these systems into balance. Also, we have seen significant improvement in some individuals when they have been treated with the NAET technique (see Glossary) for various hormones and/or neurotransmitters.

• There are so many techniques and healing modalities available that it can be overwhelming to decide where to begin or where to turn next. It is important to listen to your own intuition in this regard. However, fear, doubt, confusion, and preconceived notions can certainly affect the ability to receive clear guidance. A cocreative relationship with a practitioner you trust is very valuable, especially when you are frightened and ill. Seek out people who can help you tune into your own wisdom, be it through kinesiology, dowsing, expanding your channel, interpreting dreams, or simply learning to trust that inner voice.

• It is essential to have a sense of hope and the belief that you can get well. Seek out professionals and support groups that offer that philosophy. A profound healing on the physical, mental, emotional, and spiritual levels can be truly magical, and there need be no limits.

• Ask Spirit for help—be it through God, the Divine Mother, your Godself, angels, the Universe, or any other concept of the Divine that you feel connected to. We live in a freewill zone, which means beings in the other dimensions cannot interfere with our freewill choice. They can only intervene when invited to do so. They are waiting for you to ask, and they WILL respond. However, it may not be in the way you are expecting, so expect the unexpected, pay attention, and be open to receive. A book may fall off a shelf; you may get an unusual or timely phone call; you may run into a particular person who ignites a process for you . . .

• People become ill for a variety of reasons. Some people have experiences of amazing, spontaneous healings through prayer or as a result of going to a healer. If, however, on a soul level you are trying to learn something, you are not likely to be one of those people. We have come to view energetic healing, not necessarily as a curative treatment, but often rather as a tool that allows clients to experience their bodies in a balanced state, to feel their energetic bodies, and to become conscious of how different thoughts and experiences affect them. This awareness then offers the opportunity for them to engage in self-healing techniques, and, if they so choose, to eventually alter their programmed responses to life and its multitude of varied experiences. Patricia's first MariEL treatment was a good example of this.

• If you find that no matter what you do, it only helps for a limited period of time, or you are only able to progress to a certain level of wellness, we suggest exploring the emotional and spiritual connection of your illness. We often find that people think they are already doing this, and are unable to see where they are separated from parts of themselves. We *thought* we were in touch with this process until we talked with Vywamus!

• It was immensely helpful to us to shift our focus from the external cause of a symptom to observing our internal process, connecting that to the symptom, and honoring the communication from our bodies. This was a critical step in letting go of seeing ourselves as victims of our environment.

• Symptoms may not go away all at once. Healing all the different parts of self takes time. Patricia experienced a cyclic recurrence of symptoms such as flare-ups of Candida, digestive problems, severe menstrual pain, chancre sores, herpes-like lesions, headaches, depression, exhaustion, and muscle and joint pain. These recurrences were episodic. As her healing progressed, the time between flare-ups became longer and longer; the flare-ups themselves became progressively shorter, until they have all but ceased to occur. At this point, she is usually able to respond to communications from her body in the moment, and any problems that arise are easily remedied.

• When any illness has manifested in the physical body, it needs to be treated at the physical level. However, the trauma to the psyche can be very deep when one finds oneself in such a vulnerable state. It is easy to fall into a fear of being in the world (Vywamus is telling us the fear already existed, and our souls have chosen to magnify the pattern so we can deal with it and make a choice to be here). To stop re-creating the problem once the physical body and the nervous system have healed may take a lot of attention to what thoughts dominate your psyche and a purposeful shift to focusing on seeing yourself well.

• The more you are willing to accept and play with the notion that your thoughts create your reality, the more you can move out of the victim role and into the role of creator. Eventually you realize that it is only your fears, doubts, and judgments that keep you from creating what you want in your life. It can be a lot of fun to realize the level of power you actually do have.

• In your process of focusing on the wellness you are intending to create, allow yourself to focus on what will bring you joy. If your expectation is that if you get well, your only choice is to return to a job or an environment that did not nurture you—and, perhaps, even contributed in some way to your illness—your motivation to get well is probably compromised. This is a point where the illness offers yet another opportunity for transformation. You are rebuilding your life. Create one that nurtures your inner child and feeds your soul—a life that you love!

# Appendix V

## *Resources*

This is a list of practitioners, channels, mail-order companies, and information resources we found particularly helpful in our healing process. As has been stated several times throughout this book, we strongly encourage people to attune to their inner knowing and connect with those practitioners and resources which are right for them wherever they are in their healing.

Acupressure Institute
1533 Shattuck St., Berkeley, CA 94709
(510) 845-1059
We found the various exercise series in their book *Acu-Yoga* to be gentle and balancing.

Pat Balzer, M.S. & Halsey Snow, Ph.D.—Vywamus Channels
The Vywamus Center
1 Blackstrap Rd., Cumberland, ME 04021
(201) 797-6106; fax (201) 829-6373

The Bio-Integral Resource Center
P.O. Box 7414, Berkeley, CA 94707
(415) 524-2567
A nonprofit corporation that provides practical information on the least toxic methods for managing pests.

Mary Elizabeth Jochmans
P.O. Box 4230, Blaine, WA 98231-4230
(360) 371-3134

The Living Source
P.O. Box 20155, Waco, TX 76702-0155
(817) 776-4878
A mail-order company that carries products for chemically sensitive
people.

Dr. Devi Nambudripad
6714 Beach Blvd., Buena Park, CA 90621
(714) 523-0800; fax (714) 523-3068

Steven Rochlitz
Human Ecology Balancing Sciences, Inc.
P.O. Box 737, Mahopac, NY 10541
(914) 228-4162; fax (914) 228-4615

Sheila Simon, R.N.—Vywamus Channel
The Vywamus Connection
53 Richardson Rd., North Leverett, MA 01054
(413) 367-0356

Adriana Van Stralen, RPP
93 Main St./South Mall, Andover, MA 01810
(508) 474-4234

# Glossary

AYURVEDA: System of health care and preventive medicine from India dating back thousands of years. The root words from Sanskrit mean "science of life."

BARRIER CLOTH: A tightly woven cotton cloth used predominantly to cover pillows and mattresses. The extremely tight weave protects bedding from dust mites and minimizes odors emitting from the bedding and pillows.

BIO-TRON PROJECTOR: A device invented by the late Dan C. Roehm, M.D., which projects biotrons, fundamental energizing particles, into the user's energy field with a variety of effects.

*CANDIDA ALBICANS:* A single-celled yeast which normally resides in the human body in the mucous membranes of the digestive tract and the vagina. Ideally, it coexists in a balance with other friendly microorganisms.

CANDIDIASIS: An imbalance of microorganisms in the body in which *Candida Albicans* has proliferated. Yeast overgrowth in the gut is believed by many alternative practitioners to be a cause of food and environmental allergies, nutritional deficiencies, frequent infections, and various forms of chronic illness.

CHAKRAS: Energy centers in the body. Traditionally, the seven major chakras have been located at the subtle level along the spine with correlations to different endocrine glands and nerve plexi. The chakras serve as transducers to step-down the higher-vibrational energy of Spirit into form on the physical plane. Various teachers have said that as part of the planetary changes now underway, humans are evolving to, or reactivating, a system of twelve major chakras which will ground them more deeply into the Earth and connect them more fully to the cosmos.

CHANNEL: To receive and disseminate information and energy from a nonphysical plane; also, a person who receives and disseminates information from a nonphysical plane.

CHARCOAL MASK: A face mask, usually made of cotton, which holds an insert of charcoal tightly packed and covered with cotton. Worn by chemically sensitive people to filter out chemicals, odors, pollens, and dust to help minimize reactions.

CHRONIC FATIGUE SYNDROME: A complex illness characterized by incapacitating fatigue, neurological problems, and a constellation of other symptoms. It is known by a variety of other names, including Chronic Fatigue Immune Dysfunction Syndrome (CFIDS), M.E. (Myalgic Encephalomyelitis), chronic Epstein-Barr virus, and others. A significant number of people with chronic fatigue syndrome show evidence of having environmental illness.

CHIEF NEGATIVE FEATURE: In the Michael Teachings, this is the main obstacle to achieving one's goal in a lifetime, the primary stumbling block we have set up so that we can learn about the characteristics and consequences of that particular feature. The seven chief negative features are self-deprecation, arrogance, self-destruction, greed, martyrdom, impatience, and stubbornness. (For more on these features, read *Transforming Your Dragons* by José Stevens.)

CLEARING: A releasing of energies from the body, often of various emotions and/or physical sensations, which results in greater integration of the individual's mental body, emotional body, physical body, and spirit body.

DENNY FOIL: A vapor barrier used in construction. It consists of a thick paper coated with foil on both sides.

DIATOMACEOUS EARTH: Powder of ground-up fossil material used to kill insects such as fleas; works by poking holes in the insect's skeleton causing it to die of dehydration.

DISCONNECT: Used in this book to refer to individuals' separation from parts of themselves.

DIVINE MOTHER: Spiritual eminence in female form, the presence who answers our prayers. She has love for humans and protects them and promotes harmony and peace. When humans sincerely aspire for happiness, harmony, peace, and light, it is the Divine Mother who helps. When humans on Earth are afflicted with difficulties, it is the Divine Mother who relieves suffering and lifts them up.

ENTITY: In the Michael Teachings, a sentient being, or oversoul, comprised of 800 to 1200 individual souls.

ENVIRONMENTAL ILLNESS (E.I.): A state of imbalance in which people experience a heightened sensitivity to chemicals, foods, and inhalants. They react to exposures to minute levels of chemicals and can exhibit a broad range of symptoms that affect two or more systems in the body. In the extreme form this disorder makes people unable to leave their homes. Also referred to by many other names, including Multiple Chemical Sensitivity Syndrome (MCS), Total Allergy Syndrome, and 20th-Century Disease.

ESSENCE: Soul, Spirit, higher self.

ETHERIC: A frequency band just beyond the physical which serves as the template for all physical reality.

FRAGMENT: A part of one's self which is in a separated state.

FRAGMENTATION: Separation of a part or parts of self from one's wholeness.

FUTON: A mattress, usually made of cotton matting and a cotton cover (sometimes surrounded by foam), fashioned after mattresses used in Japan.

GAPPING: Fragmenting, separating.

GROUNDING: Connecting one's energies to the Earth; being energetically present in one's body.

HEBS: The acronym for Human Ecology Balancing Sciences.

HELIOS: Ra, the Sun God.

HUMAN ECOLOGY BALANCING SCIENCES: The system devised by the physicist, Steven Rochlitz, which advocates the use of energy balancing and ecological interventions in the treatment of environmental illness, Candida, and related disorders.

INHALANTS: A term in allergy medicine which refers to particles in the air such as dust, mold, and pollens, which, when inhaled, trigger an allergic reaction.

KINESIOLOGY: Muscle testing. The study of using changes in muscle strength to learn from the body which factors are strengthening it and which are weakening it. In recent years kinesiology has been integrated into a wide range of disciplines to enhance well-being and performance. Some areas of note include health care, education, psychology, sports, and ecology. See Appendix II for additional information.

KUNDALINI YOGA: A system of yoga that utilizes exercise, breathing, the science of sound and rhythm, and the power of the mind to help individuals live in accordance with their inner aims and to fulfill their destiny.

MACROBIOTIC DIET: A philosophy of food and health which was brought to the United States by the Japanese scholar, George Oshawa. It incorporates the Oriental philosophy of Yin and Yang. This diet is based on whole grains, beans, soy products, and sea and land vegetables.

MariEL: A form of energy/spiritual healing developed by Ethel Lombardi in 1983. MariEL promotes health at all levels by releasing energetic blocks, including cellular memories of traumatic experiences.

MCS: Acronym for Multiple Chemical Sensitivity Syndrome.

META-INTEGRATION: An advanced set of energy-balancing exercises developed by Steven Rochlitz.

MICHAEL: A nonphysical being consisting of one thousand souls who have completed their work on Earth and who continue to serve humanity by sharing information and wisdom from the mid-causal plane. Michael communicates through a variety of channels.

MID-CAUSAL PLANE: The mid-portion of one of seven levels of experience created by God, the Tao, or the Atman, for evolutionary purposes. The seven planes include the following: Physical, Astral, Causal, Akashic, Mental, Messianic, Buddhaic.

MULTIPLE CHEMICAL SENSITIVITIES: Another name for environmental illness.

MUSCLE TESTING: See KINESIOLOGY.

NAMBUDRIPAD ALLERGY ELIMINATION TECHNIQUE (NAET): A method for healing allergies which views allergic symptoms as being caused when an allergen shuts down energy pathways in the body. Treatment involves reactivating the affected energy pathways while the person holds the allergen in his or her energy field.

OPEN TO CHANNEL: Connect to one's higher self, teachers, and guides.

OUTGAS: The emission of gases that occurs during the aging and degradation of a material. Some degree of outgasing is seen in most of the humanmade materials produced in the last fifty years. This outgasing accounts for a large amount of indoor air pollution.

OZONE: A triatomic form of oxygen, formed naturally in the upper atmosphere or which can be generated by a machine. Ozone is used to eradicate mold and to neutralize chemicals.

OZONE MACHINE: A device used to generate ozone.

POLARITY THERAPY: A comprehensive approach to health based on the premise that balancing the flow of energy in the body provides a foundation for health. Polarity therapy was founded by Randolph Stone, D.O., D.C. Practitioners use gentle touch and guidance in diet, exercise, and self-awareness to help clients balance their energy flow and thereby support a return to health.

PYRETHRUM: An insecticide consisting of the dried heads of chrysan-themums.

QI GONG or CHI GONG: Ancient Chinese system working with the breath, the mind, and body movement to increase the body's energy and to promote health.

REFLECTION: Used in this book to refer to the process by which all of physical reality, including one's physical body, gives information about unconsciously held thoughts and beliefs.

ROTATION DIET: A diet often recommended for the treatment of food allergies in which foods are classified into families and the foods from each family are eaten at specific intervals, usually every fourth day. The rationale is that it takes three days after ingesting a food to which one is allergic to stop reacting to it. Therefore, if allergy-caus-ing foods are eaten only every fourth day, the level of reactivity is greatly reduced.

SELF-DEPRECATION: The chief negative feature in which a person assumes he or she has low self-worth.

SHAMAN: A priest/healer who has gone through a near-death experi-ence and a period of training to develop his or her abilities. This per-son is then able to access alternative realities to assist others in their healing.

SIKH: An adherent of a monotheistic religion of India founded in approx-imately A.D. 1500 by Guru Nanak. He was a social reformer who taught that all humanity is one family, all religions are equal, and all people are equal.

SOURCE: God, Universal Consciousness.

SUPER CLEAN: A concentrated liquid cleaner free of perfumes and harsh chemicals, used by people with environmental illness.

TIBETAN PURIFICATION CHANT: A chant used to purify the various elements within the body and the surrounding environment.

TIBETAN OVERTONE CHANTING: The use of vocal harmonics in self-created healing sounds as chanted by the Gyuto and Gyume monks. Listening to these sounds can have a profound effect on balancing and healing the body.

TONING: The process of using vowel sounds to bring balance to the body by restoring harmonic patterns.

TOUCH FOR HEALTH: System of energy-balancing techniques developed by John Thie, D.C., and described in his book, *Touch for Health*. He aimed at making the benefits of kinesiology and energy balancing more generally available.

TURPENES: Chemical compounds found in turpentine. Sources of turpenes include pine trees and cut grass.

VYWAMUS: A Master Teacher who has come to the Earth at this time to assist with the transformational process currently underway.

# Bibliography

Ashford, N.A., and C.S. Miller. *Chemical Exposures: Low Levels and High Stakes*. New York: Van Nostrand Reinhold, 1991.

Bamfort, Nick. *M.E. (Chronic Fatigue Syndrome) and the Healer Within*. Woodstock, NY: Amethyst Books, 1993.

Bell, I.R., C.S. Miller, and G. Schwartz. "An Olfactory Limbic Model of Multiple Chemical Sensitivity Syndrome: Possible Relationships to Kindling and Affective Spectrum Disorders." *Biological Psychiatry* 32 (1992): pp. 218-242.

Chopra, Deepak. *Magical Mind Magical Body*. Chicago: Nightengale-Conant Corporation, 1990. (tape set)

_____. *Quantum Healing: Exploring the Frontiers of Mind/Body Medicine*. New York: Bantam Books, 1990.

_____. *Unconditional Life: Mastering the Forces that Shape Personal Reality*. New York: Bantam Books, 1991.

Cullen, Mark R., ed. "Workers with Multiple Chemical Sensitivities." *Occupational Medicine: State of the Art Reviews* 2 (4): 1987.

DeRohan, Ceanne. *Right Use of Will: Healing and Evolving the Emotional Body*. Santa Fe, NM: Four Winds Publications, 1986.

_____. *Original Cause: The Unseen Role of Denial*. Santa Fe, NM: Four Winds Publications, 1986.

_____. *Original Cause: The Reflection that Lost Will Has to Give*. Santa Fe, NM: Four Winds Publications, 1987.

Goldman, Jonathan. *Healing Sounds: The Power of Harmonics*. Rockport, MA: Element, Inc., 1992.

Goldstein, Jay A. *Chronic Fatigue Syndromes: The Limbic Hypothesis*. Binghamton, NY: The Haworth Medical Press, 1993.

Green, Nancy Sokol. *Poisoning Our Children: Surviving in a Toxic World*. Chicago: The Noble Press, Inc., 1991.

Hay, Louise. *You Can Heal Your Life*. Carson, CA: Hay House, 1987.

Hileman, Bette. "Multiple Chemical Sensitivity." *Chemical & Engineering News* 69 (29) (1991): pp. 26-42.

Jochmans, Mary Elizabeth. *Changing Cords of Fear into Chords of Love*. Blaine, WA: Alma Tara Publishing.

Lewith, G., J. Kenyon, and D. Dowson. *Allergy and Intolerance: A Complete Guide to Environmental Medicine*. London: Green Print, 1992.

Marciniak, Barbara. *Bringers of the Dawn: Teachings from the Pleiadians*. Santa Fe, NM: Bear & Company, 1992.

_____. *Earth: Pleiadian Keys to the Living Library*. Santa Fe, NM: Bear & Company, 1995.

McFadden, Steven. *Ancient Voices, Current Affairs: The Legend of the Rainbow Warriors*. Santa Fe, NM: Bear & Company, 1992.

Nambudripad, Devi S. *Say Goodbye to Illness*. Buena Park, CA: Delta Publishing Co., 1993.

Rochlitz, Steven. *Allergies and Candida with the Physicist's Rapid Solution*. Mahopac, NY: Human Ecology Balancing Sciences, Inc., 1991.

Roehm, Dan. "Introducing the Biotron Era." Ft. Lauderdale, FL: Biotron Connection, 1991. (pamphlet)

Rogers, Sherry A. *The E.I. Syndrome: An Rx for Environmental Illness*. Syracuse, NY: Prestige Publishing, 1986.

_____. *You Are What You Ate: An Rx for the Resistant Diseases of the 21st Century*. Syracuse, NY: Prestige Publishing, 1988.

_____. *Tired or Toxic?: A Blueprint for Health*. Syracuse, NY: Prestige Publishing, 1990.

Sams, Jamie, and David Carson. *Medicine Cards: The Discovery of Power Through the Ways of Animals*. Santa Fe, NM: Bear & Co., 1988.

Sattilaro, Anthony J. *Recalled by Life*. New York: Avon, 1984.

Serinus, Jason, ed. *Psychoimmunity & the Healing Process: A Holistic Approach to Immunity & AIDS*. Berkeley: Celestial Arts, 1988.

Silva, José, and R.B. Stone. *You the Healer*. Tiburon, CA: H. J. Kramer, Inc., 1989.

Stevens, José. *Transforming Your Dragons: How to Turn Fear Patterns into Personal Power*. Santa Fe, NM: Bear & Co., 1994.

Sui, Choa Kok. *Pranic Healing*. York Beach: Samuel Weiser, 1990.

Tate, Nicholas. *The Sick Building Syndrome.* Far Hills, NJ: New Horizon Press, 1994.

Thie, John, D.C. *Touch for Health.* Marina del Rey, CA: DeVorss & Co., 1979.

Wright, Machaelle Small. *Behaving As If the God In All Life Mattered.* Jeffersonton, VA: Perelandra, Ltd., 1987.

_____. M A P : *The Co-Creative White Brotherhood Medical Assistance Program.* Jeffersonton, VA: Perelandra, Ltd., 1990.

_____. *Dancing in the Shadows of the Moon.* Jeffersonton, VA: Perelandra, Ltd., 1995.

# About the Authors

Robert C. Sampson, Jr., is a Phi Beta Kappa graduate of Yale with a medical degree from the University of Pennsylvania. He specialized in psychiatry at the University of Michigan and in child psychiatry at the New England Medical Center. A diplomate of the American Board of Psychiatry and Neurology, he is a fellow of the American Academy of Child and Adolescent Psychiatry. For sixteen years he was a psychiatric consultant to the Massachusetts Rehabilitation Commission's Disability Determination Services. He is listed in *Who's Who in the East.*

For more than twenty years, Dr. Sampson has studied alternative approaches to healing and integrated them into his professional work. He graduated from the New England School of Acupuncture in 1984. From 1985 to 1987 he was medical director of the Sino-U.S. Qi Gong Health Sciences Development Center's United States office. In connection with that program, he was an instructor in psychiatry at Harvard Medical School from 1987 to 1990. He has written several papers, including "Healing in the Treatment of Modern Medicine," which appeared in *Somatics*, Autumn 1978, and "Qi Gong Health Sciences and an Integrated Approach to the Treatment of AIDS," which was presented at a 1987 conference held in Beijing. He has spoken to a wide variety of audiences on accessing inner resources for healing.

Patricia Hughes received her Baccalaureate in Nursing from Oakland University in Rochester, Michigan, in 1978. She spent the next fourteen years working as a staff nurse in intensive care and coronary intensive care units, including four years at Boston's Harvard-affiliated Beth Israel Hospital. She was an avid fan of aerobic exercise and worked as a certified aerobics instructor for one year before she became ill. In 1984, at age thirty, she began to experience a gradual, serious decline in her health. In

1987, after several allopathic doctors were unable to help her, she was diagnosed with environmental illness. As the hospital atmosphere became more difficult for her to tolerate, she reduced her hours there and started working part-time in a holistic office setting.

Robert met Patricia in 1989. One year later, exposure to new carpet triggered his sudden onset of environmental illness. Then began their journey together in a desperate search for a way to heal themselves. After months battling for survival, they defied the conventional wisdom that environmental illness would always limit their lives. They overcame their sensitivities and attained greater health than they had known before.

Robert and Patricia now live in New Hampshire and have a private practice in Andover, Massachusetts. They work with others seeking to heal themselves of environmental illness, chronic fatigue syndrome, allergies, and related disorders. They have a strong commitment to sharing with others what they have learned about healing environmental illness and its relationship to the planetary transformation now in progress.

Robert and Patricia are available for consultations and can be reached by mail at the following address:

Patricia Hughes, B.S.N., & Robert Sampson, M.D.
P.O. Box 5071
Andover, MA 01810

They can be reached by phone at (508) 474-9009.